BODY BY SIMONE

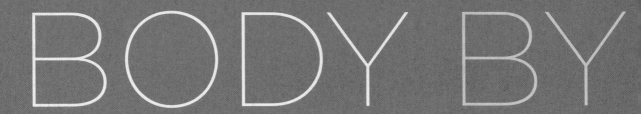

BODY BY

HARPER WAVE

An Imprint of HarperCollins*Publishers*
www.harperwave.com

SIMONE

The 8-Week
Total Body Makeover Plan

SIMONE DE LA RUE

with Lara McGlashan

BODY BY SIMONE. Copyright © 2014 by Simone De La Rue. Foreword copyright © by Grace Hightower De Niro. All rights reserved. Printed in the United States of America. No part of this book may be used or reproduced in any manner whatsoever without written permission except in the case of brief quotations embodied in critical articles and reviews. For information, address HarperCollins Publishers, 10 East 53rd Street, New York, NY 10022.

HarperCollins books may be purchased for educational, business, or sales promotional use. For information, please e-mail the Special Markets Department at SPsales@harpercollins.com.

FIRST EDITION

BOOK DESIGN BY SHUBHANI SARKAR

Library of Congress Cataloging-in-Publication Data
De La Rue, Simone.
  Body by Simone : the 8-week total-body-makeover plan / Simone De La Rue.
    pages cm
  ISBN 978-0-06-226935-5
  1. Exercise for women. 2. Physical fitness for women. 3. Women—Health and hygiene. 4. Dance. 5. Cardiovascular fitness. I. Title.
  GV482.D4 2014
  613.7'045—dc23
                              2013039888

14 15 16 17 18 OV/QGT 10 9 8 7 6 5 4 3 2 1

For my mum.

And all those who
dare to dream.

Contents

Setting the Stage

Learning the Choreography

Fuel Your Fire

The Performance

Foreword

by Grace Hightower De Niro

When I came to Simone three years ago, I was heavier than I had ever been in my life. Like so many women, I kept putting everything and everyone else in front of me. I was busy to a fault, taking care of my husband and kids, and was preoccupied with everyone's needs except my own. I kept saying, "I will exercise tomorrow, I'll get more sleep tomorrow, I'll eat better tomorrow." And before I knew it I didn't recognize myself. Now, I am a curvaceous woman, and I know I can never be a Skinny Minnie, but I wanted to put everything neatly in the right places for my body and my frame. I wanted to lose weight and tone up; and, moreover, I wanted to *feel* better.

I had been doing regular gym workouts, but there was no motivation or incentive or encouragement—the trainers just stood there, counting off repetitions, and I was really tired of machines. I believe your body *is* a machine, and that is what you should be moving and working, not some metal pulleys and handles. And I have always loved dancing, so when a friend suggested Simone and her dance-based program, of course I was excited. This could be the workout I was looking for!

And it was. Simmy's personality was so amazingly upbeat and kind, and I immediately connected with her. She literally did the workout alongside me, encouraging me and motivating me. She was so full of energy that it was contagious, and after I powered through the first session I was hungry for more.

But regardless of Simone's bubbly attitude, for a long while I did not want to look at myself in the mirror; I realized that I had not been loyal and true to myself for some time. I had always been an athlete and had kept my weight within a certain range, but I had gone way past my comfort zone. I avoided my reflection and was disappointed in myself that I had allowed this to happen.

But Simmy was so patient and so encouraging, I really started to enjoy the workouts. I gradually looked in the mirror more and more and found that I liked to watch how I was moving. I began to feel the love I was giving to myself, and the more I felt the love, the more I could look at myself in the mirror. Soon enough I saw myself transforming. Of course there was the physical transformation: I lost weight, and my arms, legs, waist, and shoulders got very toned. My posture improved tremendously and I was able to wear the fabulous clothes I loved and had so much enjoyed wearing before. But beyond the physical, there was also a significant mental transformation for me as well. I reconnected with myself, and began to appreciate my body for what it could do and how it was shaped. I loved to watch it move and groove and took pride in my curves and tone.

These days I cannot go more than a day without doing a Body By Simone workout. No, seriously, I can't! It is my drug and my sanity. This program is freeing and rejuvenating and simply fabulous.

And now this transformative program is available to everyone, right here in these pages. This book is for you—mom, wife, girlfriend, and businesswoman. BBS is something you can do for yourself that will make you look and feel better. Eventually, like me, you will get to the point where you are empowered; you will be loving, loyal, and true to yourself, because you are incredible, and that is all that matters. Simone and her program can help get you there. You just have to open the book and go for it.

Best,

Grace

A Letter from Simone

I began dancing when I was three. I don't know why I was compelled to do so—perhaps I saw a tutu or some blush-pink ballet shoes in a shop and decided that I needed to wear them; perhaps it was something deeper. Who knows the mind of a child? Thankfully, my mother indulged me, and I began taking classes immediately after I voiced my desire.

Dance became my life. I lived it, breathed it, and was totally immersed in it to the point that I *was* dance. I remember so vividly how it made me feel—joyful and free and intensely alive. Every day after school when other kids would have playdates or parties, I was at ballet. Or tap. Or jazz. When I got my first pair of pointe shoes at age thirteen, I was so excited that I tucked them into bed with me and slept with them! I still remember the feel of that bright pink satin, so smooth and shiny and perfect. Sewing on the ribbons was a religious act, and putting the shoes on my feet transported me to heaven.

While many kids grow out of activities, my dedication to dance only grew stronger as I aged. My high school friends longed for Johnny Depp, but my locker was plastered with photographs of Mikhail Baryshnikov. (Years later, when I finally got to meet him, I was too awed to even speak. I am rarely starstruck, but he left me at a loss for words!)

At age eighteen I auditioned for the Australian company of *Cats* on a whim and landed the part of the White Cat. From that point on, I became a musical-theater girl, and spent years touring with various shows in Germany, Asia, London's West End, and Australia. I finally wound up in New York, dancing on Broadway. I spent countless hours learning, rehearsing, performing, and then doing it all again the next day. I was in heaven. I was doing what I loved and loving what I did.

While I watched many of my friends and colleagues become sidelined by injuries over the years, I stayed consistently healthy despite the grueling schedule. It was not luck, and I wasn't shrouded in some sort of injury-repellent force field. Rather it was my pre- and post-performance routines and rituals that kept injury at bay. Early in my career I began practicing Pilates and yoga and studied human anatomy. I created my own unique movements and exercises based on what I'd learned, and I did them without fail before and after my rehearsals and shows. This routine kept me injury free, flexing and strengthening my muscles and joints in healing ways, while simultaneously developing a core of steel. As a happy side effect, this routine also gave me a very fit physique: I was lean, strong, and in peak cardio condition.

Once I retired from performing, I began a career in personal training and used the routines I had devised while I was a performer to help my clients achieve results. I found that my method, which uses mostly body weight and a little resistance in the form of bands and small weights, worked as fantastically for them as it had for me. They soon developed lean, lithe, toned bodies.

In addition to their physical transformations, I also noticed that many of my clients began standing up straighter, looking themselves in the eye in the mirror and connecting to themselves in the present moment. This was something I had not been expecting, but time and again, I saw women switch from averting their eyes from their reflection to engaging with themselves and watching their bodies closely, carefully, and thoughtfully as they moved and danced. These women were learning to love themselves and their bodies while they were getting in shape, which sent me over the moon with happiness. I absolutely *love* that what started for me as an injury-prevention plan has since turned into the ultimate girl-power program, something that women can use to transform their bodies and their attitudes all at once.

Today, I no longer have the desire to step onstage or hear the thunderous roar of an audience that was my lifeblood for so long. Instead, I live to see that joy and self-recognition in a class full of women doing a dance cardio workout, or the pride and confidence that radiates from a client as she reaches her fitness goals. These things inspire me more than performing ever could, and I hope that I can now reach you, my reader, in this way, too.

I sincerely hope you enjoy reading this book as much as I enjoyed writing it for you, and that you use it to learn and grow physically and mentally to become the best possible you. Share it with friends and loved ones and become wonderful role models for your children. Make exercise and healthy eating part of your life and teach those around you what you've learned. Most of all, I hope this book can help you reconnect with the joy we all experience as children when we move freely and unabashedly, letting the music move our hearts and souls. Dance with abandon, and the world will dance with you.

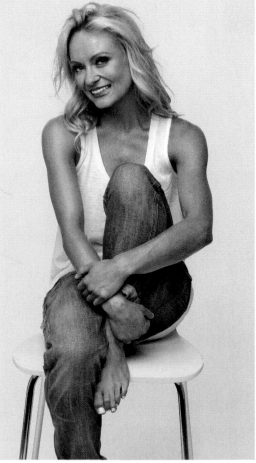

XOXO

Simone

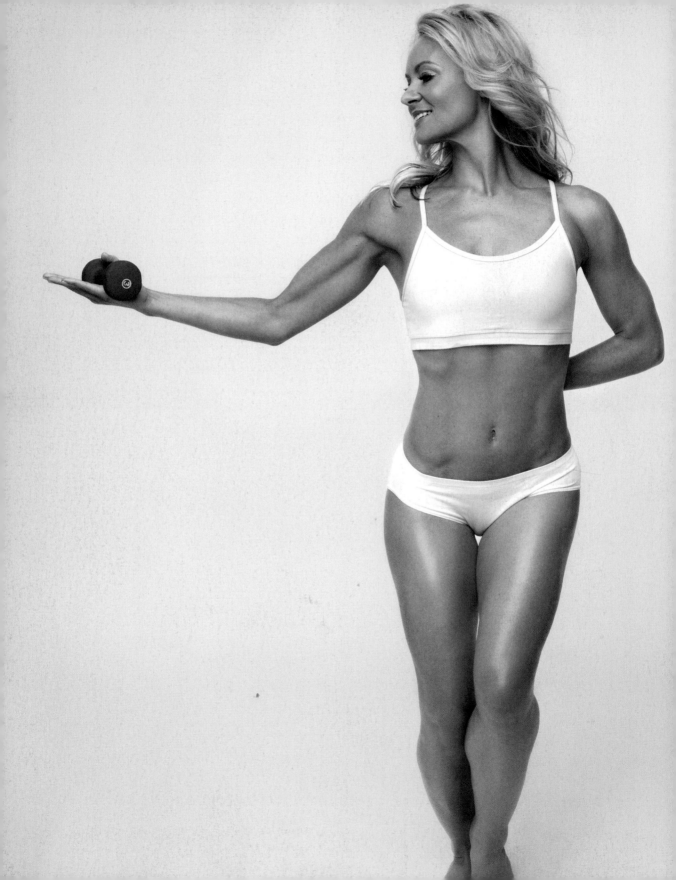

Setting the Stage

Chapter 1
The BBS Playbill

Nobody cares if you can't dance well. Just get up and dance.
Great dancers are great because of their passion.

—MARTHA GRAHAM

About BBS

The Body By Simone program, or BBS, is not a quick fix; it is a life-style. This might sound like a cliché, but it's true. I would never tell you to work out six times a week for two hours a day to get results . . . or promise that you'll lose ten pounds in a week if you do as I say. That's crazy talk! And it's not sustainable. With BBS, you will learn how to make exercise and healthy eating a way of life instead of drudgery. I'll give you the tools you'll need, and if you put in the time and effort, you'll come out the other side healthier, happier, and stronger.

The fundamental elements of the BBS exercise program are based in the movements of dance, but this does not mean you have to be a dancer to do them. Anyone of any age and ability can do this program, I promise! Dancing is a whole-body activity, and with that in mind I created workouts that use all your muscles from head to toe each time you exercise. Each workout is broken down into its most basic components, and I will take you through them, literally step-by-step, so that even someone with two left feet can easily understand them! And for those who have danced before, I hope to reconnect you to that joy and freedom you remember from your days in-studio. It is still there inside of you, waiting to come out. Release it and remember!

The BBS program offers two kinds of workouts, and you will be doing both of them to get the best results possible:

THE BBS STRENGTH WORKOUTS challenge all your muscles, from head to toe, with graceful, powerful motions. You'll utilize your body weight and light resistance from bands or hand weights to create long, lean muscle mass.

THE BBS CARDIO WORKOUTS will get your heart pumping, burn fat, and give you energy with easy-to-follow dance and jump-rope routines. Dancing has many benefits, not the least of which is fun! It also teaches coordination, balance, and concentration. And jumping rope is a high-intensity exercise you can do anywhere, anytime.

Both the Strength and the Cardio workouts are included in each of the three different levels of programs in this book. I created beginner, intermediate, and advanced programs so that you can find a workout that's right for you, one that doesn't feel overwhelming but keeps you on your toes (so to speak). No matter what your age, ability, or starting point, there is a level that is right for you in here.

My program also includes guidelines for healthy eating, along with some delicious recipes to try, which can greatly enhance your results. Good nutrition is important not only for weight loss but also for maintaining energy and concentration throughout the day. I don't believe in starving yourself or counting every little calorie you put in your mouth. Food should be about nourishment, energy, and flavor! The recipes I share in this book combine healthy ingredients with flavorful herbs and spices and are the perfect complement to the BBS program.

Great Expectations

What kind of results should you expect to see at the end of this program? More than pounds lost, I tell my clients that they will notice inches lost. You'll definitely shrink all over! Your clothes will fit differently and your friends and family will notice your transformation. Everything "sucks in"—your waist, hips, and thighs. Your arms and shoulders will become defined and strong, and your gorgeous bum will become even more gorgeous. Your legs will be lean and toned. Your whole body will become less soft, more firm, and you'll have loads of energy to spare.

You'll also find the joy in moving your body. Whether you were once an athlete or dancer, or are a complete beginner to exercise, you can and will connect to your body and your spirit through movement. You'll rediscover what it is to be active and powerful and will learn to appreciate what your body can do. I've seen some incredible metamorphoses in my classroom that I never thought possible, with clients and friends alike: women who were once bound up and constrained, letting it all hang out and being free. What an incredible change!

Because of these experiences, I strongly believe that exercise can empower you mentally. The sheer act of taking control of your health and fitness, of becoming stronger in your body, builds mental strength. When my clients are sweating in my studio, everything about them becomes more powerful and more gorgeous—their aura, their personality, their very being. If they can do it, so can you!

So what are you waiting for? Let's get started!

Q&A

QUESTION: I add muscle easily. Will your Strength Program make me bulky?

ANSWER: No! Using your body weight and light resistance will create long, lean, shapely muscles. My Strength Workouts focus on high repetitions to sculpt the ideal dancer's body.

QUESTION: Can I do both the jump rope and the dance workouts for my Cardio?

ANSWER: Sure! Just don't do them both on the same day. Choose one or the other, or alternate between the two during the course of a week so you don't overdo it.

QUESTION: I have a big event (wedding, high school reunion, etc.) coming up—will this program help me fit into my dress?

ANSWER: If you follow the program, yes, you will notice a physical transformation. So you might well fit into that dress, depending, of course, on how many inches you have to lose. And I can promise that your arms, shoulders, back, and legs will look stronger and sexier in any dress you choose; you'll stand up straighter; and you'll exude confidence. Plus, you'll be able to outmove everyone else on the dance floor!

QUESTION: I have not exercised for years. Can I still do this program?

ANSWER: Absolutely. Anyone at any level can do BBS. Start at Level I. Follow the routine slowly and deliberately. Take your time and make sure you stretch afterward to help you recover. After you feel comfortable with the routine in Level I, you can challenge yourself with Level II. Or you may want to stay in Level I for the entire program—that's totally fine! Everyone progresses at different rates. Just do what is best for you and your body.

QUESTION: How many days a week should I exercise?

ANSWER: I recommend exercising 3–6 days a week, depending on your fitness level. See page 44 for a more thorough breakdown of the levels and recommended training times, as well as some notes on the importance of rest days.

QUESTION: I have never been a good dancer and am scared of looking silly. Can I really do your program?

ANSWER: First of all, just go ahead and look silly! No one is watching you, right? Dance your brains out, and don't worry about what people think of you. Secondly, you can definitely do these routines. I break each movement down into its simplest units, with accompanying photos, so it's easy to follow. If you need another visual aid, go to my website at www.bodybysimone.com and check out our videos. I've got you covered!

Chapter 2
A Reflection of You

The first time I started choreographing was in the dark, in my living room, with the lights completely out, to some popular music on the radio. I put the radio on full blast and I started moving. I didn't know what it looked like. I didn't want to see it . . . I had to start in the dark.

—JUDITH JAMISON, *DANCING SPIRIT: AN AUTOBIOGRAPHY*

The Mirror and Me

As a dancer, I have been looking at myself in the mirror for years and years. I didn't think much of it; it was just part of my life. But once I became a trainer, I discovered that many women have trouble with this. It's difficult for them to look at themselves and connect with and accept who they are and how they look. They are so critical of and uncomfortable with their physical body that oftentimes they avoid looking at their reflection altogether.

In addition to the amazing benefits of weight loss and increased muscle tone, my program also offers you the tools for inner transformation. I want you to learn to appreciate yourself and your incredible, beautiful body. I want you to be able to look in the mirror and feel strong and proud, no matter what your station in life, no matter what your job, no matter what your current weight or body shape. To smile at your own reflection and hold your head high is a gift. And there is nothing more powerful, more sexy, more unstoppable than a woman who is proud of who she is.

Staring at yourself in the mirror might feel a little awkward at first, but give it time. As I've mentioned, I've worked with many women who are mirror-averse but who eventually are able to connect with that image in front of them in a powerful way. To help them on that journey, I developed an exercise I call Mirror Minutes that allows you to connect to yourself on a deeper level.

Mirror Minutes

Stand about a foot away from a mirror and look into your eyes. No, not the floor, or the coffee table, or the mole on your cheek—your eyes. Spend some time here. See yourself for who you are right now. Mentally list your attributes. Do you like your lips? Your collarbones? Your booty? Your abs? Give yourself some positive credit. Even my clients with so-called "perfect" bodies don't always see their beauty. And the truth is, there's no such thing as a perfect body—there is only a perfect version of you.

Once you've identified things you feel positive about, start moving. Look at your body in the mirror as you move. Dance is about power and beauty, about the physical blending with the ethereal. The movement of your body can impart joy and strength, and being able to appreciate that is key to letting go and connecting to the movement in a spiritual way.

You know that saying "Dance like nobody's watching"? I want that to become your mantra. Dance in the dark if you want to. Sometimes with my clients, I'll turn down the lights in the studio and watch the transformation. You can see the questions pass over their faces—am I allowed to do this? To be this? To let go and be silly, or funky, or gorgeous? But then they do, and it's incredible.

Watching yourself move in the mirror will help you connect to your body, and being connected to your body will better enable you to perform the exercises in this book with the proper form. You will gain an increased physical awareness of where you are in space and how your limbs move. All of this will make doing my workouts easier, more enjoyable, and more effective.

I know that Mirror Minutes can be challenging for some women, but it really does get easier. You will get used to studying your reflection instead of avoiding it, and as the weeks pass you'll notice the physical changes taking place with greater clarity.

At the beginning of each workout, I want you to start by doing Mirror Minutes for 5 minutes. Connect to your spirit and your soul, then begin to exercise. A good mind-set is key to a good workout!

Don't Bring Yourself Down

Women have a bad habit of bringing one another down, being critical and gossipy about each other's personalities and appearances. We do it to ourselves, too. How crazy is that? You may not even realize you're doing it, but most of us say negative things about ourselves and our bodies every day. Even those small things we say in passing—complaining about our hair or the way our jeans fit or that we're having a bad skin day—are detrimental to the way we think about ourselves over the long term.

If you are unhappy with your body, you've probably caught yourself saying or thinking something especially negative about it recently. Think back over the course of the past week—did you complain to someone else about your tummy, your hips, your thighs, your arms, your butt? Probably so. I know I catch myself doing it as well. This is not a habit that can be instantly changed, but here's an exercise to help you break it:

Choose Your Words Wisely!

Remember that old adage "Sticks and stones may break my bones but words will never hurt me"? Turns out it was wrong: There has been some interesting research done on negative words and the impact they have on the brain. For instance, one group of researchers found that the word "no" can trigger the release of dozens of stress-producing hormones in the brain, causing anxiety, interrupting logical thinking, and impairing communication! It was also found that simply showing anxious people a list of negative words for only a few seconds

The Power of Mantras

When my clients are struggling with Mirror Minutes or with any other exercises, I tell them to think of a mantra they can repeat in their heads to give them the strength to push through fear and doubt. Here are a few examples of mantras that have worked for them:

"Confidence, strength, beauty."
"I am worthy."
"I know I can, I know I can."
"This time is mine."
"I am a vision of health and beauty."

caused sleeplessness, depression, and loss of appetite. It's really incredible how a simple word can completely disrupt your whole mindset, so it's imperative to change unhealthy thought patterns. Negative thinking is self-perpetuating—meaning, the more time you spend doing it, the more likely you are to continue doing it. Let's break this cycle.

To prevent myself from being negative, I try to think about everything I am going to say before I say it, and if I feel it might be negative, I catch it before it passes my lips. I then reframe that thought, make it positive, and release it into the universe, so to speak. It's definitely a difficult exercise at first, but just as the phenomenon of negative thinking can be self-perpetuating, so, too, can positive thinking become a self-perpetuating habit.

Here's an exercise to try. On a piece of paper make two columns, one labeled "Negative" and one labeled "Positive." Each time you have a negative thought or say something negative about yourself, write it down in the "Negative" column; if you have a positive thought or say something positive about yourself, put it in the "Positive" column. At the end of the week, look over the comments in both columns. Which one has more items? If it's the Positive column, that's incredible! Keep it up! If the Negative column has more items, you've got some self-love work to do, darling.

Let's take this exercise one step further: take the negative comments from your week and tweak them to make them positive. For example, perhaps your paper reads like this:

"I can't wear skinny jeans—my thighs are too big!"
"I will never be able to wear a sleeveless dress with this arm and back fat."
"Today I feel frumpy and mushy."

Now take these negative comments and turn them into positive ones! This might take a little bit of thinking, but it will be worth the time.

"I love the way my lower body looks in an A-line skirt!"
"I will take control of my body and health by working out consistently. By summer, I will be able to wear a sleeveless dress!"
"I'm not feeling my best today, but I know I'll get back on track tomorrow."

See how that works? The more love and encouragement you can give yourself, both mentally and physically, the quicker your body and attitude will turn around.

When you see yourself in a more positive light, it's a lot easier to make positive changes in your life.

Self-Love Checklist

Self-love is often a challenge. Not sure where to start? Go down this checklist of body parts. Find something you like about each part and write it down. Refer to it often when you find yourself spiraling into negativity!

eyes	smile	fingers	booty
brows	hair	fingernails	back
cheekbones	neck	bust	thighs
face	arms	waist	calves
nose	shoulders	hips	feet
lips	hands	belly	toes

No-No Words

There are some words that I suggest you simply eliminate from your vocabulary. See if you can find an alternative word or phrase to replace these self-defeating ones and use those instead!

NO-NO WORDS	REPLACEMENT WORDS
Example: Can't	Example: Can!
Won't	_____

Unable	_____
Should	_____
Powerless	_____
Weak	_____
Tired	_____
Sluggish	_____
Fat	_____
Defeated	_____
Ugly	_____

The Ideal Body

I grew up in the ballet world, where being thin was expected, and even forced upon you. We were measured and weighed every week, and I witnessed numerous friends develop eating disorders that left them injured and ill. That is a horrible way to live, and I am thankful every day that I had a mother who made it a priority to take care of my body and my spirit and prevent me from getting sucked into that obsessive, destructive cycle.

The pressures of the dance world offer an extreme example. But the truth is that most women today are obsessed with achieving a certain body type. Whether you want to look like a celebrity or someone you know, this kind of wishful thinking inevitably leads to disappointment and frustration, especially if you simply don't possess the body type of the person you want to look like.

I can assure you that your body type role models are really just like you—they have fat days and thin days, days when they wake up with zits or a bloated belly. They have days when they think they look old or tired or frumpy. But what they do have that you don't is a good stylist, a transformative makeup artist, and a photographer with a retouching computer program to correct those flaws and make them look perfect!

My point here is that no one is perfect, not even those who appear to be so. They are human, like you, and have flaws, like you. Once you realize this, you're one step ahead of the curve. The trick is to embrace your flaws and imperfections. Once you've accepted that your body type is unique to you, you can start to think about the areas you'd like to target for improvement.

The best way to start this process is to look at your body shape objectively. Stand in front of a mirror (yes, again!) and look at your frame. Are you broad in the shoulders and narrow in the waist? Do you have curvy legs and thighs? No curves at all? Don't be critical of what you see, just observe and note.

Now look at the following body-type composites and see where you fit in. You probably won't fit perfectly into any one category, so just find the ones that most closely match your physique.

Body-Type Composites

Apple Shapes

WHAT: Apple shapes are characterized by a larger bust, broader shoulders, narrower hips, and a less-defined waist.

WHO: Celebrities like Elizabeth Hurley, Kelly Osbourne, Angelina Jolie, Catherine Zeta-Jones.

HOW: Apple types tend to carry more body fat in their midsections. Targeting the core is essential for this type. I suggest doing the core exercises of your strength program first so you have plenty of energy to devote to them. Apples can also focus on building their legs to counterbalance their broad shoulders. My favorite move for Apples is Planks (page 70).

Pear Shapes

WHAT: Pear-shaped ladies are wider through the hips, thighs, and bum, have narrower shoulders, and a smaller bust.

WHO: Celebrities like Kim Kardashian, Jennifer Lopez, Shakira, Kelly Clarkson.

HOW: Pear-shaped women carry their extra weight in their glutes and thighs. They should focus on building their shoulders and arms to counterbalance their naturally larger lower half. My favorite move for Pears is the Double Curl and Reach (page 87).

Hourglass Figures

WHAT: Hourglass body types have a bust and hips of roughly the same size, a well-defined waist, and shapely legs.

WHO: Celebrities like Salma Hayek, Scarlett Johansson, Sofía Vergara, Jennifer Hudson.

HOW: An hourglass shape usually has a pretty even distribution of weight throughout her body and should focus on building the upper and lower bodies equally. My favorite move for Hourglass gals is the Window Washer (page 98).

Tomboy Types

WHAT: This type is characterized by a straight, noncurvy waist and hips, a small bust, and an athletic frame.

WHO: Celebrities like Naomi Watts, Kate Hudson, Cameron Diaz, Keira Knightley.

HOW: Tomboy women can add curves by training the shoulders, glutes, and legs. They can also add shape to their waist by doing exercises that hit the obliques and transverse abdominal, and building their butts with plenty of squats and lunges. My favorite move for Tomboy types is the Double Towel Slider (page 98).

Which of these shapes is the most like your body? With this perspective in mind, take some time and reassess your fitness goals. Are your expectations or desires achievable given the overall shape you were born with? This is important, because if you're coveting the physique of Kate Hudson when you yourself are more like Shakira, you're probably going to be frustrated with your results. And it's difficult to appreciate your achievements when you're hoping for something completely different. Own the beautiful genetics you've got and make them work for you.

No matter what your type is, BBS will help you become the best version of it. Genetics are one thing, but you *can* improve things like body composition (your muscle-to-fat ratio), the definition and tone in your limbs and core, and your energy level. You can trim inches from your waist, arms, hips, and legs. You can even add shape and breadth to narrow shoulders and improve stooping posture.

Take some time to formulate your goals with these things in mind. Once you've decided on your goals, write them down. We'll discuss goal-making in detail later on, but you can get a head start now. Writing it down in black and white makes it powerful and real.

Role Call

My role models growing up were always dancers, not because of their bodies but because of their talent. This was fortunate, because, as a result, I was more obsessed with being powerful and athletic and strong than with being rail-thin. I admired their artistic gifts, and the bodies that helped them translate that gift in beautiful ways—not how they looked in a dress on the red carpet.

In fact, my ultimate role model was Mikhail Baryshnikov—certainly not some-one whose body I could achieve! I watched his movie *White Nights* over and over again, and I admired his strength and grace, and of course his ability to do eleven pirouettes in a row and make it look effortless. He moved with such ease and fluidity, but could also bound and jump like an elite athlete. I was fascinated with his true-life story of defecting from the Soviet Union to the U.S.A. Anyone who is so driven by their passion that they would risk losing their family and their past forever is amaz-ing to me. He literally came from nothing and worked his way to fame with blood, sweat, and tears. In my eyes he is the greatest ballet dancer of the twentieth century, and one of my all-time most-admired people.

Jane Fonda is another one of my role models. The fact that she is seventy-five years old and looks the way she does absolutely floors me. I mean, come on! When you look at her, you can't make any excuses about being too old or too tired to work out. Jane Fonda literally paved the way for women to be fit and healthy and to love their bodies. She was one of the first women ever to do a workout video, and thou-sands of people around the world followed her programs and remember her iconic leg warmers and striped leotards. To this day, a lot of her exercises remain some of the most effective for toning the lower body, and I even incorporate some of her moves into my studio classes as a tribute to her genius. I also think she is a great political activist who helps amplify the voices of women. I admire her tenacity and strength when it comes to issues she is passionate about.

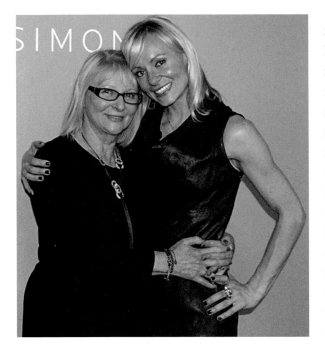

And, of course, there is my ultimate role model: my mum. She was a single mother, but I never lacked for anything. She supported me no matter what I wanted to do, and she is the reason I was able to pursue my dreams. My mum came to every one of my dance auditions, and sat outside on the cold, hard chairs, waiting for me to finish my ballet exams. She picked me up after school and drove me to dance every day without fail. She did a million jobs to help fund my career, and I owe everything I am to her, including my person: her strength, generosity, and gentleness are traits I always admired and hope to emulate in my own life. She taught me to chase my dreams, but to be kind along the way. If I am half the woman she is, I will be very, very lucky.

Today when I speak to young women about their role models, they often name the faces we all see on the covers of magazines. That's fine, if they admire those people on the inside and out, but often it seems like our role models are chosen more for their beauty or their style than for their brains. Think about the people you count as your role models, and ask yourself what it is about them that inspires you. And if you don't have role models—it's time to identify some! It might be an athlete or a celebrity, a politician or a powerful businesswoman, or, as with me, it could be a family member. Try to choose someone based on her mental attributes as well as her physical ones. Admire her for her accomplishments and achievements and list things you like about her in a broader sense than simply the corporeal. Just as it's important to have goals in your life and in your fitness, it's also important to have role models who inspire you to reach those goals.

Chapter 3
Warming Up

When I dance I cannot judge, I cannot hate, I cannot separate myself from life. I can only be joyful and whole. That is why I dance.

—HANS BOS

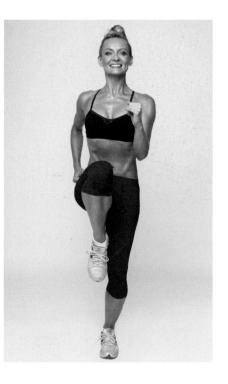

Being prepared is paramount to success in anything you do. If you have all the tools you need before you start, you'll have no excuse not to continue. So the first order of business is everyone's favorite part: shopping! Even though many of my exercises don't require any equipment at all, there are some basics that increase the intensity of the workout and will help you to achieve results. Just about everything is available online or in sporting goods stores, so do a few Internet searches to find the best deals.

Equipment

Resistance Bands

Resistance bands come in a variety of styles: some have handles at either end while others are simply long pieces of elastic sheeting. All kinds of bands will work for my routines, so choose the style you like best and go with it. Bands also come in a variety of "weights": the thicker the band, the more challenging it is to use. I suggest getting a few different bands; as you get stronger you'll want a little more "weight"! Cost: $5–$10.

Hand Weights

Dumbbells are affordable and easy to store. I suggest using a pair of 2-, 3-, or 5-pound weights for my routines. I also like the Reebok Thumblock Wrist Weights, nifty little things that Velcro onto your hands so you don't have to worry about dropping them. Cost: $5–$10.

Pilates Ball

This soft, squishy ball is about 12 inches in diameter and is used, in various capacities, in all my workouts. It does not have much weight; rather it's used for balance, style, and form. Cost: about $10.

Water Bottle

Hydration is essential to keep your muscles and body working properly. I suggest investing in a PBA-free water bottle and carrying it with you everywhere. You can never drink enough water! Cost: about $10.

My client Lucy Damon and her husband, Matt, turned me on to a charity called Water.org. Nearly a billion people in the world are without safe drinking water, but we can help! With each purchase of a Water.org water bottle, $10 goes toward bringing safe water and sanitation to people in developing nations. These water bottles are available everywhere online (I even offer the link on my website!).

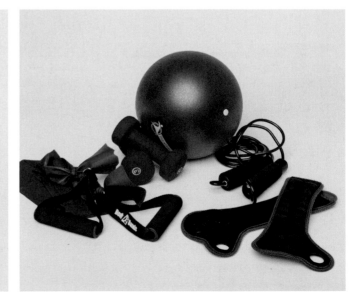

Hand Towel

Grab any old towel from your linen closet and you're good to go—I can promise you that you're going to need it for these workouts!

NOTE: The Level III: Soloist Strength Workout requires a second hand towel for a series of exercises, so make sure to have two—one for your face and one for your feet.

Yoga Mat (Optional)

If you're working out on a hard surface I suggest using a yoga mat to cushion your bones and joints, especially when doing your floor work. Cost: $8–$30, depending on thickness and brand.

Jump Rope (Optional)

I have created a jump-rope routine for each Cardio level to add some variety to your program. You don't have to do the jump-rope workout, but if you do, I suggest investing in a plastic speed rope, like the kind used by boxers, or a beaded rope that has a little weight to make it turn more easily. Follow the directions on the packaging to make the rope the correct length for you. Cost: $3–$30.

Music, Man!

What is dance without music? The right music can make a workout inspiring and uplifting, and motivate you to keep going. I don't know about you, but music can literally change my mood: if I am feeling blue or low-energy, the right song can pull me out of my funk and get me off the sofa. I'm sure you know what I'm talking about (especially if you drive on a daily basis . . . cranking up the right radio song changes everything!).

You can work out to practically any music, but I strongly suggest you do my workouts to your favorite beats. When putting together a playlist, choose songs that energize you and encourage you to work hard. Rap, R&B, pop, even classical—any or all these genres can work if you find them motivating.

For the Strength Workouts, I suggest selecting slower songs with a strong beat. They should all have a similar pace (about 128 beats per minute—or BPM—if you're savvy about counting music). Here's a sample playlist I love to use with my clients for Strength Workouts:

"Run Run Run," by Phoenix

"I Know What You Want," by Busta Rhymes and Mariah Carey

"The Way Life Used to Be," by Snoop Dogg

"Changes," by 2Pac

"Butterfly," by Crazy Town

"Man in the Mirror," by Michael Jackson

"Freedom," by George Michael

"Signs," by Snoop Dogg (with Charlie Wilson and Justin Timberlake)

"Last Night a D.J. Saved My Life," by Indeep

"Get Up," by 50 Cent

Counting

Counting music is not as hard as you'd think! Here's how it breaks down:

A MEASURE, OR BAR, in music is a collection of beats, four or eight, for example. (The inside joke in the dancers' community is that we only know how to count to eight, since that is the most common measure in dance!)

FINDING THE BEAT is tricky for some people, so I always suggest listening for the drums, since they are usually easy to distinguish from the rest of the instruments. Once you've found the beat, listen to the song a few times. Count how many times you hear that beat in fifteen seconds. Multiply that by four to get the number of beats per minute. The BPM number determines the tempo of a song: the higher the BPM, the faster the song, and the lower the BPM, the slower the song.

WHEN PUTTING TOGETHER A PLAYLIST, try to find songs that closely match one another in terms of BPM, or go onto iTunes to find songs that already have the BPM listed. You can also buy apps that alter the tempo of a song, so if you really want to add a tune to your playlist and it's too fast or too slow, tweak it with an app!

For the Cardio Workouts, choose faster-paced songs, which fall in around 132 to 138 beats per minute, just fast enough to give you a good workout without hindering your form. Here is a playlist I use for my classes that everyone loves:

"Somebody That I Used to Know (Tiesto Remix)," by Gotye

"Ready Steady Go," by Oakenfold

"Arosa (Original Mix)," by Andrea Oliva

"Don't Stop Dancing (Extended Mix)," by Kaskade 7 EDX

"Barbra Streisand (HK Mix)," by Weekend Millionaires

"Feel So Close (Radio Edit)," by Calvin Harris

"Let's Go" (Radio Edit), by Calvin Harris (with Ne-Yo)

"Day N' Nite (Crookers Remix)," by Kid Cudi

"I'm the Ish" (Remix featuring Kanye West)," by DJ Class

"Don't You Worry Child (Radio Edit)," by Swedish House Mafia

If you're not into making your own playlist, there are tons of websites where you can buy ready-made workout music, such as iTunes, in their Fitness and Workout section. Spotify is also a great way to access millions of jams for free, so you can sample what you like.

> Want to hear what I'm playing in my class right now? Go to www .bodybysimone.com and check out my playlist of the week!

Making a Space

Okay, I know that not everyone who buys this book has a studio in her garage with a sprung dance floor. But you don't need a fancy studio space to create a great environment for your workouts. Here are some suggestions for commandeering a little corner of the world for yourself:

* Wherever you choose to create your workout space, give yourself plenty of legroom. Slide tables and chairs out of the way, pick up any toys, books, magazines, or other things lying around. Then give it a test run: walk around in a large circle. Kick forward, backward, and sideways. Did you hit anything? If not, perfect! You've got enough room to work out!

- Put your weights, bands, Pilates ball, water bottle, and anything else workout-related in a box or basket, and store it in a corner of your workout space. That way everything is in one place, ready and waiting, and you'll never have to waste time looking for things.
- Prop a full-length mirror against a nearby wall so you can see yourself clearly. Correct form is important, for both safety and effectiveness, as is watching and connecting with yourself in the mirror as you do the exercises.
- If you're working out on a hard surface, I strongly suggest using a yoga mat so you don't bang or bruise your knees and hips when doing floor moves.
- Once you've established your space, sit quietly on the floor and close your eyes. Visualize yourself using this space while transforming into the best version of yourself possible. Imagine yourself exercising, dancing, and smiling here in this space. Feel your heart pumping and your energy soaring. Feel the joy you're going to experience over the next eight weeks, then open your eyes. Now you're ready to start.

Dress for Success

You know that fabulous feeling you get when you're wearing a great outfit? I know that when I'm dressed in a way I love, I feel powerful, strong, confident. You can have that same feeling when you're working out, as well. Here are some suggestions to help get you outfitted properly for your workouts:

- Wear comfortable, form-fitting clothing that's not too baggy. You'll want to be able to see your muscles working and make sure your form is correct.
- Choose athletic shoes that offer support in all directions, such as cross trainers or flexible dance shoes.
- Invest in a supportive sports bra. This makes all the difference in the world in terms of comfort, whether you're well-endowed or not, especially during the Cardio Workouts.
- Wear clothes that make you feel good about yourself. If you love your arms, wear a sports tank. If you adore your calves, get some capri pants. As you go

through the program, allow yourself to splurge on a new top or bottom to show off your sexy new muscles. When you see the progress in the mirror, it will help keep you motivated.

Attitude Adjustment

The most important equipment of all when you're working out is your attitude. Go into each session with an open mind and heart. By carving out time for yourself and your health, you are investing in your future in the most important way. There will be days when you don't want to exercise, and I get that. Here's a little trick to get you going: tell yourself you'll just do ten minutes. That's it—just start moving and sweating, and if you're still not feeling it, you can stop. But I guarantee once you start you'll immediately feel better and will finish the whole workout. I've done my best to create fun, exciting workouts that you can look forward to, so let yourself enjoy this time, and have a little fun.

Skip the Scale

I have absolutely no idea how much I weigh, and I don't particularly care. So many people are addicted to their scales, religiously weighing themselves every day. For these women, a pound one way or another on the scale can be the difference between a great day and a dismal one, which is a really unhealthy way to exist.

Your "weight" is nothing more than a measure of how hard gravity is working to pull your body toward the center of the earth. It does not take into account your muscle mass, your fat mass, how much you ate that day, or how much water you're retaining. I know that I typically feel a little bloated and heavier when I'm approaching my cycle— hormonal fluctuations can have a real influence on your weight. But I also know that it's not permanent, and in a week I'll be back to normal. So instead of hopping on the scale, I suggest using photos, clothing fit, and measurements to gauge your progress.

When it comes to photos—we take "selfies" all the time. With friends, at restaurants, on vacation, texted or posted for the world to see. How about putting that technology to use for your health and snapping a few photos of your body in the here and now? Wear whatever athletic clothing makes you feel good and take at least three photos of yourself from the front, side, and back. Then take a candid look at these photos. Even if you don't love what you see, remember—no negative talk allowed. Just use these as your baseline so that you can check in as you progress and see how your body is changing.

Did you know . . .

That muscle weighs more than fat, but is more compact and takes up less space? Therefore you can "weigh" more and wear a smaller dress size if you have more muscle! My Strength Workouts will help you gain some of this lean, dense tissue, and the Cardio Workouts will help you shed the bulkier fat.

Clothing fit is another great way to monitor your progress. Clothes that are snug now should gradually become looser. You know those skinny jeans you've got in your closet? Bring them out. Put them on. How do they fit? Consider taking a photograph wearing those, too. Write down how they feel on your body. Eight weeks from now, you're going to put them on again and see how they look and feel.

I also recommend that you measure yourself with a cloth tape measure. Wrap it around yourself to measure the circumference of your upper arms, thighs, hips, waist, and bust. Be sure to measure around the thickest part of each of these areas, and write the results down. At the end of this journey you'll repeat this process and see how far you've come.

Chapter 4
Waiting
in the Wings

I do not try to dance better than anyone else. I only try to
dance better than myself.

—MIKHAIL BARYSHNIKOV

There are two more key things I want to discuss before you get
started on your program: goal setting and journaling. These activities will help you
stay mindful of your intention and keep you accountable.

Setting goals is an important part of anything we do in life. If we want to be
successful, we first have to define what success looks like. When it comes to your
fitness routine, setting a goal that you want to achieve by the end of these next eight
weeks will help you stick to your program. The key to setting your goals is to make
sure that they are *specific* and *achievable*. For instance, wanting to lose thirty pounds
by the end of the month is probably not a realistic, achievable goal. (Plus, it requires
that you get on a scale, which is not something I advocate!) Setting far-fetched goals
sets you up for failure: When you don't reach them, you'll be bummed out and less
motivated to keep going.

On the other hand, wanting to "be stronger" is a nice idea for a goal, but it's
not very specific—how do you know when you've achieved that? It's important to
set goals that are measurable so that you know when you've reached them, and can

celebrate your success. A better goal might be: "I want to gain enough strength in my arms to do five push-ups." That's a specific and achievable goal.

Here are some other examples of goals that are specific and achievable. Note that not all of them are about toning up or losing weight—because connecting your mind and body and nourishing yourself with good foods is about so much more than that.

- I will fit into my skinny jeans.
- I will drop one or two dress sizes.
- I will work out five times a week.
- I will lose inches on my waist, hips, and bust.
- I will have more energy and a better attitude.
- I will improve my endurance so that I can run a 5K.
- I will lower my cholesterol and blood pressure.

Take some time to think about your purpose for doing this program and what you'd like to get out of it. Then write down your goals. I know that if I have a goal, I like to write it big and bold on a piece of paper and hang it where I'll see it several times a day, like in my office or on my bathroom mirror. It's a nice little reminder and helps me stick to my plan on days when I'm veering off course.

I also encourage you to make little goals that can help you achieve your big goal. Reaching smaller goals is very encouraging and can help keep you on track. These can be weekly or even daily goals. Here are some ideas:

- I will drink at least eight glasses of water today.
- I will bring my lunch to work this week instead of eating out.
- I will get up thirty minutes earlier to do my workout in the morning once a week.
- I will choose more whole foods than processed ones today.
- I will cook myself healthy meals at least four nights a week.
- I will really push myself during the strength workouts today.
- I will leave work in time to get home and do my workout tonight.

Ink It

I am a big advocate of keeping a food and exercise journal or log. It keeps you on track with your program by making you accountable. And just like with any other to-do list, it's very satisfying to write down your accomplishments at the end of the day. I always recommend journaling to my clients to help ensure their success.

Your journal can be anything from a notebook to a fancy app on your phone— whatever is handy and convenient for you. The more consistent you are with your notes, the more useful it will be. At the end of each week, review your log and see what you can learn. It will be crystal clear where you've succeeded and where you've struggled. For example, when you look at your log you might notice that you have trouble working out on Friday evenings, because you want to relax with your family or meet friends for dinner. So why not switch your Friday workouts to the morning? Likewise you might see that you struggle to make good food choices at breakfast when you're tempted by bagels or doughnuts at the office, so you can make a decision to eat a healthy breakfast at home before heading out each morning. Your journal is a tool that can help you create the best strategy to meet your goals. (Write your goals in your journal as well so they're within easy reach.)

Your journal will also help you notice trends that are less obvious, such as when you have the most energy, how your workouts help relieve stress, and how your mental outlook is affected by your fitness choices. At the end of the program, you'll gain a lot of insight from these kinds of notes.

I suggest that you log your workouts (what you did, and for how long), your nutrition (what you ate, how much, and when), and your overall mental outlook (stressed, high-energy, tired, sharp, unfocused, etc.) each day. All of these elements are important when you're trying to reach your goals, and they are all closely related to one another. Writing them down helps you see how they connect to form your bigger picture of health.

Workout Notes

Once you've got the basics down, here are a few other notes you might want to include about your workout:

- HOW YOU FELT BEFORE THE WORKOUT. Your frame of mind can make or break your workout session, so it's important to note your attitude going in.
- THE TIME YOU WORKED OUT. At certain times of the day you'll have more energy than others. Noting the time you did your workout will help you recognize when you are in the best physical condition to exercise. Note the correlation between how you felt before and after your session in order to decide whether the time you're exercising is right for you.
- HOW YOU FELT AFTERWARD. I am a firm believer that moving your body can help reset your brain. Many people find exercise to be a great stress relief, although there will also be days when you feel bogged down and tired. Note how you feel, good or bad.
- ANYTHING ELSE YOU THINK IS IMPORTANT TO MENTION. Life happens, and sometimes you'll be distracted by work, family, or stress. All of these things can affect your workout experience. Jot down a few notes about what is happening in your day, and how it's affected the way your body is feeling.

Nutrition Notes

Keeping track of what you eat is important for a few reasons. First of all, it often nips bad choices in the bud—you might think twice before eating that cookie if you know you're going to have to write it down. Second, looking at a record of what you've eaten within the context of how you felt before and afterward can also help you recognize eating patterns, or even food sensitivities or allergies. For example, you might notice that you crave sugary foods around 4 p.m., when you're in an energy slump. Or that after eating dairy foods like milk or cheese you feel bloated and sleepy. A food log is a great way to gain insight into why you're eating what you're eating—and how that food is helping or hurting you.

In addition to the basics (what you ate, how much, and when), here are a few things to consider noting in your journal:

- HOW YOU FELT PHYSICALLY AND EMOTIONALLY BEFORE EATING. How did your body feel? Were you starving? Tired? Not even that hungry? Thirsty? What about your mind—were you in a good mood? Stressed out and grumpy? On autopilot and grabbing something on the go?

- HOW YOU FELT PHYSICALLY AND EMOTIONALLY AFTER EATING. Were you full and satisfied, or were you still hungry? Did you still have cravings, or did they fade away? Were you angry at yourself for bingeing on chips, or proud of yourself for choosing broccoli over fries?
- HOW MUCH WATER YOU DRANK. Water not only hydrates you, it also transports nutrients throughout your body and helps to naturally detoxify your system by flushing out toxins and waste. I recommend drinking at least 8–10 glasses a day, more if possible, to keep your body working properly. Each time you drink a glass of water, mark it in your journal.

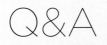

QUESTION: I am not big into journaling. Do I have to do this to succeed with BBS?

ANSWER: You don't *have* to do it, but I strongly encourage you to give it a try. There are so many benefits to journaling that it would be a shame not to explore it. Tell you what: try it for a week and see how it goes. If you still hate it, fine, don't do it anymore. But I bet once you start you will get addicted.

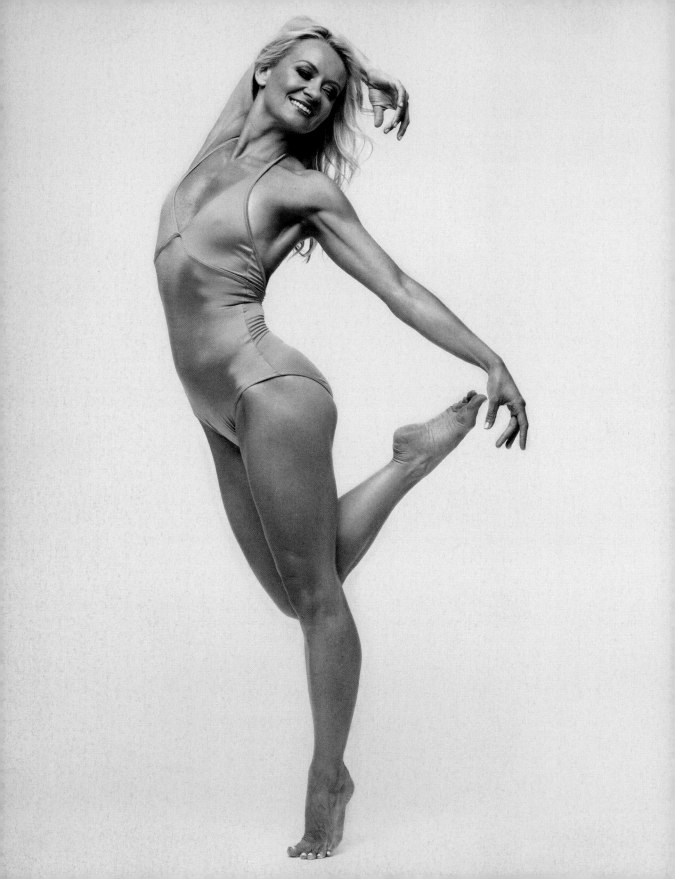

Learning the Choreography

Chapter 5

Onstage

To dance is to reach for a word that doesn't exist, to sing the heartsong of a thousand generations, to feel the meaning of a moment in time.

—BETH JONES

I spent decades engaging each muscle group in my body every single day. Every time I went to the studio to rehearse, every time I stepped onstage to perform—I used every muscle I had, head to toe. It's this knowledge and experience that has shaped the way I work out, and how I train my clients. Each time you exercise using the BBS program you'll work all the muscles in your body—that's what makes this program a total-body workout. Targeting multiple muscle groups in one session is a highly effective method for shaping and defining muscle tone *and* burning fat at the same time—not to mention, making the best use of your limited workout time!

Beyond offering a total-body experience, my style of training has also been called the "girlfriend" workout (by the *New York Times*, in fact!) because women love doing it, and they often bring their friends to class so they can all do it together. In addition to reaching your fitness goals, I want you to experience that sense of fun and light-heartedness, to feel a renewed connection to your body, and to gain the confidence that comes with being a strong, healthy woman.

The Workouts

As I mentioned earlier, I developed three different levels of the program, so that anyone at any ability can achieve meaningful results.

LEVEL I: CORPS DE BALLET. This is the beginner level. If you're not someone who exercises regularly, or if you're coming back to exercise after a hiatus, an injury, or pregnancy, start off at Level I. You can always increase the intensity and go up to Level II if you feel that you're beyond the basics, but I'd rather have you work your way up than start out feeling over your head.

LEVEL II: SOLOIST. This is the intermediate level. If you exercise moderately 2–3 days a week and have the endurance to complete at least 45 minutes of intense cardio, this is the level for you.

LEVEL III: PRINCIPAL. This is the advanced level. When I teach classes at my studio, I usually train my students at the Principal level. These workouts are tough, but they produce results. If you're someone who currently exercises at least 4 days a week, give it a whirl. If it's too much right away, try Level II for a few weeks and come back to Level III when you're ready.

Some of you might want to complete the full 8-week cycle at one level, while others will work their way up a level (or even two!) as the weeks progress. The important thing is to gauge whether your workout is still challenging you—once it becomes routine, or too easy, it's time to increase the intensity or change things up. You can even mix and match your workouts as you gain strength and ability—maybe you're comfortable at Level II but not quite ready for a full week of Level III. So try alternating your workouts—Level II one day, Level III the next. Eventually, you'll find yourself choosing more Level III days than Level II days. There are no hard-and-fast rules about how you should do these workouts. I only ask that you continue to push yourself so you can reach your goals.

Be sure to check in with yourself each week. In addition to the obvious signs of progress, like how your clothes fit, how many inches you've lost, and how much you've changed from the day you took your "before" photo, review your journal to see how you *feel*. Are you sore and tired? Give yourself an extra recovery day. Are you a little bored? Challenge yourself by stealing a few moves from the next level up. Remember: these are *your* workouts. Choose the level you think best suits your abilities, go at your own pace, and have fun!

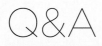

QUESTION: I used to be very athletic, but I haven't worked out much in the last several years. Where do I start?

ANSWER: Start with Level I: Corps de Ballet. This is a good place for you to test your ability while avoiding the possibility of injury that might come with going too fast too soon. Even if you've taken some time off from exercise, your body probably has something called *muscle memory*, which is the term for physiological pathways in your nervous system that result from training your body. Maybe you used to play a sport or run 10Ks. Those activities created pathways to activate specific motor units and muscle fibers to help you perform . The more you did that activity, the more those motor units fired, and the more your muscle memory was reinforced. So most likely, once your body recognizes that you're moving and grooving again, it will bounce back quickly.

Getting Started

I've designed separate Cardio and Strength workouts specifically for each level. All of the workouts should be preceded by a warm-up and followed by a cool-down as well as some stretching and flexibility training (see page 123) to maximize your performance and prevent injury. I recommend that you do the Cardio before the Strength workout in order to kick the heart rate up, but if you prefer to reverse the order, that's fine—just make sure you don't skip out on your cardio after you've worked up a sweat! You can also split up each workout into two mini-workouts, doing Cardio in the morning, for example, and Strength in the evening, as your schedule allows.

I recommend training 3–6 days a week, depending on your ability. Those new to an exercise program can start with 3 days and work up from there, whereas those of you who work out more regularly can start out at 4 or 5 days weekly. Your training schedule will be an individual thing. Be sure to take time to recover if you feel like you've been overtraining—and kick it up a notch if you feel like you've been under-training!

But one thing is certain for all levels: you have to take days off to recover. Always schedule at least one to two rest days into your workout schedule to avoid injury, low energy, and overtraining—a condition in which you exercise too much and never adequately recover. Besides putting you at a higher risk for injury, overtraining slows your metabolism, since your body is working overtime trying to heal itself and is less likely to burn body fat.

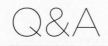

Q&A

QUESTION: I did my first workout and I am so sore! Why does everything hurt?

ANSWER: Most post-workout soreness is attributed to delayed-onset muscle soreness, or DOMS.

Even though I have been exercising for years, I still get fabulously sore from a good workout! DOMS comes from microscopic tears in your muscles that are the result of challenging them with a new form of exertion, such as dancing or lifting weights. These tears result in new muscle growth, allowing you to gain strength and endurance so that you can keep challenging yourself.

If you're new to exercise you might find that you're sore about 24 to 48 hours after your workout. This is totally normal! Your body repairs these muscle tears very quickly, especially if you're giving yourself adequate rest. Spend some time stretching, focusing on the muscles that hurt the most, and you should rebound in a few days.

The Mind-Muscle Connection

The mind-body connection is an essential underpinning of any exercise plan. Remember the Mirror Minutes we did in Chapter 2? You're going to use that same idea to connect with your muscles as you work out. Looking at yourself in the mirror as you exercise and paying attention to how your body moves and feels will ensure that you're engaging the right muscles and have proper form.

For example, the Shoulder Shaper (page 88) works the lateral deltoids, those outside shoulder muscles that look sexy in a sleeveless top. With each repetition you do, watch yourself in the mirror. See your shoulder moving as you lift your arm up and out to the side. Feel yourself engaging that muscle deliberately. Imagine it getting stronger. Watch how it looks as it contracts, and realize how powerful and beautiful a muscle can be when you work it.

Exercise and the Yummy Mummy

Years ago doctors warned pregnant women not to exercise, but these days we know better—being fit and healthy during pregnancy is beneficial to mum and baby. Exercise can elevate your mood, ease back pain, and help to prevent the health risks associated with gaining too much weight during pregnancy, such as gestational diabetes. And of course, a postpartum exercise plan can help you get back into your skinny jeans a whole lot faster and allows you to take care of yourself while in the midst of taking care of a new little person 24/7. That being said, you do have to approach exercise a bit differently during and after your pregnancy. Here are a few guidelines:

During Pregnancy

- First, clear any exercise program with your doctor. If you are a high-risk pregnancy, heed any and all advice your doctor gives you, even if it is not to exercise at all!
- Once you're past your first trimester, don't do any moves lying on your back, including abdominal work. This puts pressure on the vena cava, reducing blood flow to your head, heart, and uterus. I've included Mummy Modifica-

tions and alternate moves in my workouts. Opt for those versions if you are more than 12 weeks along.

- Avoid excessive bouncing, jumping, and hopping. Make the Cardio moves low-impact by keeping one foot on the ground, or by using my Low-Impact Tips that are scattered throughout each exercise chapter.
- Your center of gravity is changing every week, so be extra careful when doing anything that requires balance, and get up slowly from the floor to avoid dizziness and nausea.
- Listen to your body. Rest and cool down when it tells you it's tired or hot. Your blood volume doubles during pregnancy, which means you will fatigue faster and overheat more quickly than you did pre-pregnancy.
- Be especially careful when stretching post-workout, as your ligaments and joints are more flexible than normal. Don't push yourself past your normal range of motion.
- Weight loss is *not* the goal. You are working out for the health of you and your little one. Accept the changes your body is going through, and enjoy the process. It's not every day you get to grow another human being, after all!

Postpartum

- Check with your doctor and make sure you're ready before beginning an exercise program again.
- Start slowly. I recommend Level I: Corps de Ballet workouts for all postpartum mummies.
- Stick to the Low-Impact moves for a month or two to allow your body to regain some strength. After that, ease back into the regular routines.
- For women who have had C-sections: be sure to ask your doctor when it's safe to begin doing the abdominal work. Be extra gentle when doing exercises that target your abs or any moves that involve twisting and reaching. Your abs and core will need time and patience to recover.
- Cut yourself some slack. Sometimes you simply don't have the time or energy to work out—this is totally fine! Tomorrow is another day. Enjoy spending time with your baby on days when exercise is simply out of reach, and don't beat yourself up about it.

Four Kids, 200 pounds

I work with lots of women who are pre- and postpartum, but my poster child for looking fabulous after four babies is absolutely Lucy Damon. She worked with me after each of her pregnancies and each time shed 35–50 pounds.

How did we do it? Initially we focused on a lot of low-impact cardio, including dancing. Lucy is not a dancer, but I tricked her into it, and soon she was having so much fun that 45 minutes flew by! Once her doctor cleared her, we began to do abdominal and core work, then we amped up the cardio, gradually increasing the intensity as the weeks went by. We also did a lot of upper-body work using the Reebok Thumblock Wrist Weights. Lucy's favorite moves were the Level I arm series, especially the Sliders and the Swan Arms (see pages 62 and 61).

After 4–5 months of hard work, she was back in prime form, which is pretty impressive if you ask me. I always say, it took you 9 months to put the weight on, and it will take you 9 months to get it off!

The Wonderful Warm-Up

Before each and every workout, regardless of level, spend 5–10 minutes warming up. The warm-up is an important part of your routine: it readies your muscles, joints, and circulatory system for exercise, delivering blood and heat to all of the areas of your body that you're about to engage. A warm body is less likely to become injured, so don't skimp on your time spent warming up!

The idea of a warm-up is to get your body moving and your heart pumping. You can do anything you like, such as walking briskly, jogging in place, or doing a few jumping jacks or high knees. You can even just put on your favorite music and dance around the house for 5 minutes. If you plan to do your Cardio workout first, be sure you move all your limbs around and get everything ready to rock and roll before starting.

A good warm-up also gives you a mental transition to exercise mode. We have a thousand things on our minds every day, all of which can distract us from being present in our bodies for a workout. A good workout requires really being present and focusing on the physical—not the mental. Use your warm-up time to empty your mind of worries and issues. Imagine shedding your stress as you shake out your limbs. Feel your body coming to life as you move, your excitement and dedication increasing as your heart starts pumping. Inhale deeply and breathe out all of the toxic emotions of your day. At the end of ten minutes, you'll be ready to exercise with a clear mind and warm muscles.

The Cool-Down

Cooling down after your workout is just as important as warming up beforehand. It allows you to dispel heat, slow your heart rate, and relax your muscles without experiencing cramping or tightening. After you've done both the Strength and Cardio portions of your workout, spend 5–10 minutes cooling down. Keep moving gently and slowly. Breathe deeply and roll your head, neck, and shoulders to relax. Step side to side and swing your arms to shake them out. You can also take this time to do some gentle dynamic stretches before moving into your static flexibility training, as outlined in Chapter 8.

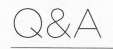

QUESTION: I have very limited time to work out. Can I skip the warm-up and cool-down?

ANSWER: I do not recommend skipping either of these important steps, since they are so beneficial to your health both mentally and physically. If you're short on time you can do an abbreviated warm-up and cool-down, but be sure to spend at least 3–5 minutes on each.

Injuries

Taking rest days, warming up and cooling down properly, and listening to your body are all effective ways to prevent injuries. But of course all exercise programs come with a risk of injury. So how do you know if you're injured, and what should you do about it if you are?

There are two kinds of injuries: acute and chronic. You will notice an acute injury right away, as it is severe or sudden—broken bones and sprains are examples. Most acute injuries are accompanied by sharp pain and swelling. These injuries require an immediate trip to the doctor, followed by the needed amount of rest to heal.

A chronic injury, on the other hand, is one that develops over time as a result of overuse, improper form, or maybe even a genetic structural abnormality in your frame. It is a pain or ache that never seems to go away, and nothing—not stretching, not rest—alleviates the pain. Conditions like tennis elbow, bursitis, and plantar fasciitis are common chronic injuries. The best course of action is to take a break from exercising and use the RICE method (see box on page 42) to alleviate your symptoms. If after several weeks you're still in pain, off to the doctor you go.

Everyone has an injury now and again. The trick is to understand it, accept it, treat it, and work around it as necessary. For instance, if you have a problem with your right knee, you can still do upper-body and core-strength moves with no problem, and, with a doctor's okay, you may be able to do the low-impact version of the Cardio workouts.

The good news is that exercise, especially resistance training, can actually help prevent injuries by strengthening the muscles around joints and ligaments to help support them. This new strength can also lead to a decrease in chronic pain and stiffness, especially in the back, neck, and shoulders.

If you're already seeing a doctor about an existing condition, ask him or her what's safe and what's off-limits. Never force yourself to do a move if it is painful, and modify the range of motion or depth of a move to suit you and your particular needs.

And no matter where or what your injury, flexibility training will be your best friend: spend at least 10–15 minutes post-workout stretching your most problematic areas. Focus on the large and small muscle groups surrounding those areas as well to improve range of motion and increase your chances of healing up faster!

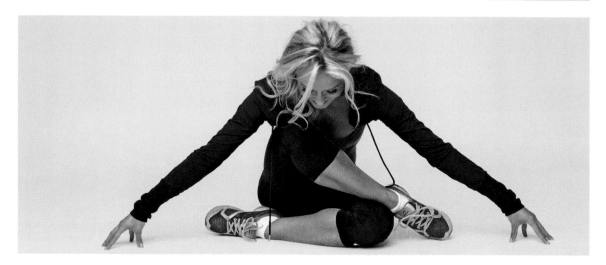

Recover with RICE

This do-at-home formula is key when you've got a minor injury:

REST the injured part for 6–8 weeks; more if necessary.

ICE the injured part in 20-minute bouts several times a day.

COMPRESS with a bandage to help reduce swelling and support the injured part.

ELEVATE the injured part above the heart to help reduce swelling.

Your body truly is a perfect machine. All your joints, muscles, ligaments, and nerves work together in specific ways to create the range of motion you need for so many different movements—from running to swimming to dancing—so it's important to keep all the cogs and wheels of your musculoskeletal system in good working order. Since everything in your body is interrelated, building strength and flexibility in one part will benefit several others in a chain reaction. For instance, strength-training the muscles of the quadriceps and hamstrings will consequently strengthen the ligaments and tendons that support and stabilize the knee, making that joint less likely to get injured. Similarly, stretching the muscles of your shoulders and upper back can release tension in the spine and neck, allowing for greater freedom of movement and reduced incidence of neck and back pain. This is why I advocate engaging in all aspects of fitness, including strength training, cardio, and flexibility. It's the best way to keep your beautiful machine in tip-top shape.

Chapter 6
The 8-Week Plan

It is health that is real wealth.

—GANDHI

I designed BBS as an 8-week program. I believe this to be a reasonable, manageable span of time in which to make significant changes in your body and adopt fitness and healthy living as a part of your life. Before we get into the workouts, I want to go over the goals and expectations for your results, week by week. Keeping track of your progress is a great way to stick to your plan and stay motivated.

REMEMBER!

You are doing a Cardio and a Strength workout every day. Don't skip either one—they are equally important! Beginning your workout with Cardio warms you up, kicks your heart rate into gear, and starts the fat-burning process, which then continues with the Strength workouts. But if on some days you want to start with Strength, or want to split your workouts into Cardio in the morning and Strength at night, that is totally fine; at the end of the day I just want you to have done both!

WEEK 1

Goal: Stay Present

This week might be a challenging one if you are new to exercise. Make it your goal to complete each and every workout to the best of your ability without getting overwhelmed or feeling defeated. Stay in the moment and know that as the weeks move forward, you will get stronger and healthier with each session. Even if some of the moves feel foreign or awkward to you at first, remember—you are teaching your body how to move using correct form and technique, which takes practice. Soon enough your muscle memory will take over!

YOUR RESULTS: You may see some weight loss in week one, but I can't promise that the changes will be dramatic just yet. I *can* promise you that you will feel more energized and comfortable in your own skin than you've felt in a long time.

NOTE: If you are doing the cleanse (see Chapter 12) in conjunction with your workouts, you may feel a bit fatigued initially. This is because your body is releasing toxins and waste, which take a few days to be eliminated from your body. Know that this is a passing feeling and it will go away shortly.

TIPS: Take your time with your strength workouts so that you learn how to do the moves correctly. This is your starting point and from here on out you will build on the foundation you're creating. Don't forget to take the time to warm up and cool down completely before and after each workout.

Week 1 Schedules

Level I: Corps de Ballet

MONDAY	TUESDAY	WEDNESDAY	THURSDAY	FRIDAY	SATURDAY	SUNDAY
CARDIO: 10 min. STRENGTH: Upper body	Off	CARDIO: 10 min. STRENGTH: Lower body	Off	CARDIO: 20 min. STRENGTH: Core	Off	Off

Level II: Soloist

MONDAY	TUESDAY	WEDNESDAY	THURSDAY	FRIDAY	SATURDAY	SUNDAY
CARDIO: 15 min. STRENGTH: Upper body	Off	CARDIO: 15 min. STRENGTH: Lower body	CARDIO: 10 min. STRENGTH: Total body	Off	CARDIO: 25 min. STRENGTH: Core	Stretch

Level III: Principal

MONDAY	TUESDAY	WEDNESDAY	THURSDAY	FRIDAY	SATURDAY	SUNDAY
CARDIO: 30 min. STRENGTH: Core	CARDIO: 20 min. STRENGTH: Upper body	CARDIO: 20 min. STRENGTH: Lower body	CARDIO: 20 min. STRENGTH: Total body	CARDIO: 30 min. STRENGTH: Core	Stretch	Off

WEEK 2

Goal: Push Through

This week you might be feeling tight, sore, and fatigued; this is completely normal. You've been asking your body to work hard, and it is changing and adapting to your demands with each workout. If you need to, do a little extra stretching this week to accelerate your recovery time and give your aching muscles some relief.

YOUR RESULTS: You may notice that your appetite is increasing—this is a good thing! It means that your metabolism is revving up and that you're burning more calories. Don't be afraid to eat: follow your gut (literally) and eat, but make sure you fuel yourself with nutritious whole foods. Resist the urge to weigh or measure yourself just yet—but do take note of how you feel as you move throughout the day and during your workouts. Do your arms feel stronger as you lift a bag of groceries? Can you do one more reps in some of your Strength moves? Your whole body should be feeling stronger and more capable.

NOTE: If you are doing the cleanse, this week you should be feeling much better, and your energy should jump dramati-

I am a big fan of foam rollers for working your sore muscles. Rolling helps improve blood circulation in your skin, muscles, and those hard-to-reach tendons, ligaments, and connective tissues. It may be a little painful at first—but rolling out your legs, back, and torso with a foam roller will help you recover from your workouts more quickly.

cally as you expel the toxins you've released as a result of your clean eating plan. You may also notice that your hair and nails have grown and your skin and eyes are glowing! Yes, these are some of the other benefits of cleansing.

TIP: Remember to eat frequent small meals and snacks throughout the day to give your metabolism the fuel it needs to repair and rebuild your hardworking muscles. And make sure your snacks are actually snack-sized: they should be about half the portion of a meal.

Week 2 Schedules

Level I: Corps de Ballet

MONDAY	TUESDAY	WEDNESDAY	THURSDAY	FRIDAY	SATURDAY	SUNDAY
CARDIO: 10 min. STRENGTH: Total body	Off	CARDIO: 20 min. STRENGTH: Upper body	Off	CARDIO: 10 min. STRENGTH: Lower body	Off	Stretch

Level II: Soloist

MONDAY	TUESDAY	WEDNESDAY	THURSDAY	FRIDAY	SATURDAY	SUNDAY
CARDIO: 15 min. STRENGTH: Total body	CARDIO: 15 min. STRENGTH: Upper body	Off	CARDIO: 15 min. STRENGTH: Lower body	Stretch	CARDIO: 25 min. STRENGTH: Total body	Off

Level III: Principal

MONDAY	TUESDAY	WEDNESDAY	THURSDAY	FRIDAY	SATURDAY	SUNDAY
CARDIO: 20 min. STRENGTH: Total body	CARDIO: 20 min. STRENGTH: Upper body	CARDIO: 20 min. STRENGTH: Lower body	CARDIO: 30 min. STRENGTH: Core	CARDIO: 20 min. STRENGTH: Total body	Off	Stretch

WEEK 3

Goal: Form Healthy Habits

It takes approximately three weeks to form (or break) a habit. By the end of this week, your new, healthy lifestyle should be a lot easier to maintain. You will find yourself looking forward to your daily exercise and might be eager to try new, healthy recipes and foods. Invest in a few good-quality cooking tools, such as a grill pan or a single-serving smoothie blender, to make preparing healthy food easier and more enjoyable.

YOUR RESULTS: You should begin to see and feel results by Week 3. Specifically, my clients often notice a difference in their waist, arms, and stomach at this point—you should feel a bit tighter and firmer all over. If you're someone who likes tangible results, get out your measuring tape and measure yourself again. Is there a difference? If so, record the results in your journal! If you're not seeing results as quickly as you want to, just remember to be patient and realistic. Rome wasn't built in a day!

TIP: Remember to write in your journal every day so you have a record of your progress. If you're not getting results as quickly as you'd like, take a look back and see where you can improve your nutrition or your exercise program.

Week 3 Schedules

Level I: Corps de Ballet

MONDAY	TUESDAY	WEDNESDAY	THURSDAY	FRIDAY	SATURDAY	SUNDAY
CARDIO: 20 min. STRENGTH: Lower body	Off	CARDIO: 10 min. STRENGTH: Upper body	Off	CARDIO: 10 min. STRENGTH: Total body	Stretch	Off

Level II: Soloist

MONDAY	TUESDAY	WEDNESDAY	THURSDAY	FRIDAY	SATURDAY	SUNDAY
CARDIO: 25 min. STRENGTH: Core	Off	CARDIO: 15 min. STRENGTH: Lower body	Stretch	CARDIO: 15 min. STRENGTH: Upper body	CARDIO: 15 min. STRENGTH: Total body	Off

Level III: Principal

MONDAY	TUESDAY	WEDNESDAY	THURSDAY	FRIDAY	SATURDAY	SUNDAY
CARDIO: 31 min. STRENGTH: Core	CARDIO: 31 min. STRENGTH: Upper body	CARDIO: 20 min. STRENGTH: Lower body & core	Stretch	CARDIO: 20 min. STRENGTH: Total body	CARDIO: 31 min. STRENGTH: Core	Off

WEEK 4

Goal: Kick It Up a Notch

You're halfway there! By the end of this week you will have completed an entire month of exercise and healthy eating. This is an amazing accomplishment and in itself should motivate you to work hard again next month. Now it's time to kick it up a notch by increasing the intensity and duration of both your Cardio and Strength workouts.

YOUR RESULTS: Your body has been developing muscle memory, so keeping your form in Strength moves and remembering the steps in the Cardio workouts should start to feel easier. You should also begin to notice definition in your arms, legs, and torso. Compare how you look now with the photos you took in Week 1. See a difference? If you're following my food plan, your cravings for sugar and caffeine should also have subsided by now, and you might notice that you now *crave* healthy food before and after a workout!

TIP: Check in with the goals you created in Chapter 4 and make sure you're on track to accomplish them. If you are on track—stay focused and keep doing what you've been doing. If you aren't, adjust your plan as needed. Now might be the time to increase the length or frequency of your workouts.

Week 4 Schedules

Level I: Corps de Ballet

MONDAY	TUESDAY	WEDNESDAY	THURSDAY	FRIDAY	SATURDAY	SUNDAY
CARDIO: 12 min. STRENGTH: Lower body	CARDIO: 12 min. STRENGTH: Total body	CARDIO: 12 min. STRENGTH: Upper body	Off	CARDIO: 12 min. STRENGTH: Total body	Off	Off

Level II: Soloist

MONDAY	TUESDAY	WEDNESDAY	THURSDAY	FRIDAY	SATURDAY	SUNDAY
CARDIO: 16 min. STRENGTH: Upper body & core	Off	CARDIO: 16 min. STRENGTH: Lower body & core	CARDIO: 16 min. STRENGTH: Total body	CARDIO: 30 min. STRENGTH: Core	Stretch	Off

MONDAY	TUESDAY	WEDNESDAY	THURSDAY	FRIDAY	SATURDAY	SUNDAY
CARDIO: 32 min.	CARDIO: 20 min.	CARDIO: 20 min.	CARDIO: 32 min.	CARDIO: 20 min.	Off	CARDIO: 20 min.
STRENGTH:	STRENGTH:	STRENGTH:	STRENGTH:	STRENGTH:		STRENGTH:
Upper body	Core	Lower body	Core	Total body		Total body

WEEK 5

Goal: Commit Anew

This is a new week in a new month and you should step it up: make your workouts more intense by using more challenging resistance bands. Increase the level of intensity in your Cardio workouts by adding extra jump-rope work. Remind yourself of your intentions and commit to four more weeks of consistent hard work. It will all be worth it.

YOUR RESULTS: This week your clothes should definitely start to feel looser—your skinny jeans should allow for some actual breathing room! Your endurance should also be increasing day by day, and you should be sleeping better.

TIP: Try out some new recipes. If you get bored with the same food over and over again, you'll be tempted to stray from the plan. Variety is the key to preventing boredom.

Week 5 Schedules

Level I: Corps de Ballet

MONDAY	TUESDAY	WEDNESDAY	THURSDAY	FRIDAY	SATURDAY	SUNDAY
CARDIO: 12 min.	Off	CARDIO: 15 min.	CARDIO: 12 min.	CARDIO: 12 min.	Stretch	Off
STRENGTH:		STRENGTH:	STRENGTH:	STRENGTH:		
Total body		Lower body & core	Total body	Upper body		

Level II: Soloist

MONDAY	TUESDAY	WEDNESDAY	THURSDAY	FRIDAY	SATURDAY	SUNDAY
CARDIO: 17 min. STRENGTH: Lower body & core	CARDIO: 17 min. STRENGTH: Total body	Off	CARDIO: 30 min. STRENGTH: Upper body & core	CARDIO: 17 min. STRENGTH: Total body	Stretch	Off

Level III: Principal

MONDAY	TUESDAY	WEDNESDAY	THURSDAY	FRIDAY	SATURDAY	SUNDAY
CARDIO: 33 min. STRENGTH: Core	CARDIO: 20 min. STRENGTH: Total body	CARDIO: 33 min. STRENGTH: Lower body & core	CARDIO: 20 min. STRENGTH: Upper body & core	Stretch	CARDIO: 20 min. STRENGTH: Total body	CARDIO: 20 min. STRENGTH: Core

WEEK 6

Goal: Don't Cheat!

Sometimes when people begin to see results they slack off a little—skipping a workout here and there, eating some pizza or cake or cookies—and all of a sudden their results are gone! This week remember to look ahead, scheduling your workouts and planning your menu for the week ahead of time, giving yourself every opportunity to succeed.

YOUR RESULTS: By now you should see results in your whole body, but especially your lower body. Your thighs will be stronger, leaner, and toned, and your booty should be perking up. These are the kinds of changes that other people will notice—so be sure to show them off at every opportunity! Instead of splurging on food or an extra rest day, why not splurge on that sexy dress that's been calling your name?

TIP: Remember to think ahead when planning your meals. I like to do my food shopping on Sunday, so that on Monday I can wake up and start my week with fresh, lovely produce at the ready.

Week 6 Schedules

Level I: Corps de Ballet

MONDAY	TUESDAY	WEDNESDAY	THURSDAY	FRIDAY	SATURDAY	SUNDAY
CARDIO: 13 min. STRENGTH: Lower body & core	Off	CARDIO: 20 min. STRENGTH: Total body	Off	CARDIO: 20 min. STRENGTH: Core	Off	CARDIO: 13 min. STRENGTH: Upper body & core

Level II: Soloist

MONDAY	TUESDAY	WEDNESDAY	THURSDAY	FRIDAY	SATURDAY	SUNDAY
CARDIO: 30 min. STRENGTH: Lower body & core	CARDIO: 18 min. STRENGTH: Upper body & core	CARDIO: 18 min. STRENGTH: Total body	CARDIO: 18 min. STRENGTH: Lower body & core	CARDIO: 18 min. STRENGTH: Upper body & core	Off	Stretch

Level III: Principal

MONDAY	TUESDAY	WEDNESDAY	THURSDAY	FRIDAY	SATURDAY	SUNDAY
CARDIO: 34 min. STRENGTH: Upper body & core	CARDIO: 20 min. STRENGTH: Total body	CARDIO: 20 min. STRENGTH: Lower body	CARDIO: 34 min. STRENGTH: Core	CARDIO: 20 min. STRENGTH: Total body	CARDIO: 34 min. STRENGTH: Core	Off

WEEK 7

Goal: Push Through with Intensity

You've only got two more weeks to go: time to get serious! Increase the number of reps you do for your Strength moves, add more songs to your Cardio playlist to make your workout longer, or up the tempo of your Cardio workouts from 130 BPM to 132 or 134. And if you haven't already progressed from Level 1 or 2, now is the time to challenge yourself. YOUR RESULTS: I am addicted to endorphins—those feel-good hormones that your body releases when it exercises—and by the end of this week you'll find that you are, too! You should be looking forward to your daily sweat session, and may even find if you don't work out you truly miss it and don't feel completely whole until you make the time to do it. By now you should feel strong, lean, powerful, and capable of doing anything you put your mind to. Oh—and you may have gone down a clothing size, too!

Week 7 Schedules

Level I: Corps de Ballet

MONDAY	TUESDAY	WEDNESDAY	THURSDAY	FRIDAY	SATURDAY	SUNDAY
CARDIO: 14 min. STRENGTH: Total body	CARDIO: 14 min. STRENGTH: Lower body & core	CARDIO: 14 min. STRENGTH: Upper body & core	Off	CARDIO: 14 min. STRENGTH: Total body	Stretch	Off

Level II: Soloist

MONDAY	TUESDAY	WEDNESDAY	THURSDAY	FRIDAY	SATURDAY	SUNDAY
CARDIO: 19 min. STRENGTH: Lower body & core	Off	CARDIO: 30 min. STRENGTH: Upper body & core	CARDIO: 19 min. STRENGTH: Total body	CARDIO: 19 min. STRENGTH: Upper body	CARDIO: 19 min. STRENGTH: Lower body & core	Off

Level III: Principal

MONDAY	TUESDAY	WEDNESDAY	THURSDAY	FRIDAY	SATURDAY	SUNDAY
CARDIO: 35 min. STRENGTH: Upper body & core	CARDIO: 20 min. STRENGTH: Total body	CARDIO: 35 min. STRENGTH: Upper body & core	CARDIO: 20 min. STRENGTH: Total body	CARDIO: 35 min. STRENGTH: Lower body & core	Off	CARDIO: 20 min. STRENGTH: Lower body

WEEK 8

Goal: End with a New Beginning

This is it—your final week! Give it all you've got in each and every workout—don't hold back! Add your own personal style to your dance moves, or even invent new choreography. Push those muscles to their limit with your Strength workouts, and make sure every movement is precise and perfect.

YOUR RESULTS: You should feel amazing at the end of this week. Get out that tape measure and your "before" picture; measure yourself again and take a new photo. You will have lost inches all over your body, and my guess is, the person you see smiling back at you from your new photo looks a lot happier and healthier than she did just 8 weeks ago. Even more important than how she looks, though, is how the woman in that picture feels—she should have more energy and confidence, and a more optimistic attitude about her health and her future. That's true beauty.

TIP: Learn to accept a compliment graciously—because you'll be getting a lot of them. If someone says, "Wow, you look amazing!" say, "Thanks! I've been working hard and it's paid off!"

Week 8 Schedules

Level I: Corps de Ballet

MONDAY	TUESDAY	WEDNESDAY	THURSDAY	FRIDAY	SATURDAY	SUNDAY
CARDIO: 25 min. STRENGTH: Total body	CARDIO: 25 min. STRENGTH: Core	CARDIO: 15 min. STRENGTH: Upper body & core	Off	CARDIO: 15 min. STRENGTH: Lower body & core	CARDIO: 15 min. STRENGTH: Total body	Off

Level II: Soloist

MONDAY	TUESDAY	WEDNESDAY	THURSDAY	FRIDAY	SATURDAY	SUNDAY
CARDIO: 30 min. STRENGTH: Total body	CARDIO: 20 min. STRENGTH: Upper body & core	Off	CARDIO: 20 min. STRENGTH: Lower body	CARDIO: 20 min. STRENGTH: Total body	CARDIO: 20 min. STRENGTH: Core	Off

Level III: Principal

MONDAY	TUESDAY	WEDNESDAY	THURSDAY	FRIDAY	SATURDAY	SUNDAY
CARDIO: 20 min. STRENGTH: Total body	CARDIO: 20 min. STRENGTH: Total body	CARDIO: 40 min. STRENGTH: Core	CARDIO: 40 min. STRENGTH: Upper body	CARDIO: 40 min. STRENGTH: Lower body	CARDIO: 20 min. STRENGTH: Total body	Off

Chapter 7
The Building of a Body

We ought to dance with rapture that we might be alive . . .
and part of the living, incarnate cosmos.

—D. H. LAWRENCE

A lot of women fear the words "strength training," but I am here to tell you that strength training is absolutely essential for women of all ages. Not only does it help you get in shape by building muscle and burning fat, it also helps to increase bone density and defend against osteoporosis. Plus, a great strength-training session is the perfect way to manage stress and let off some steam (especially those punching and kicking motions).

Muscle is more metabolically active than fat, which means that the more muscle you have on your body, the more calories you will burn, even at rest. As you begin to add more and more muscle to your frame, your metabolism will rev up and you will find that your body burns fat much more quickly than it used to. This is because your muscle cells use carbohydrates (in the form of glucose, or blood sugar) and glycogen (another kind of blood sugar, made for long-term storage) as fuel to keep your body going. When you have more muscle, it demands more of that quick fuel that you have stored, leaving your body no choice but to break down body fat to use for its metabolic functions and activities.

Style Points

The BBS program is graceful, beautiful, and powerful, and the underlying technique is derived from dance. Maintaining proper form for all of your strength-training moves is essential to getting results, so I encourage you to follow the instructions for the moves as written. But feel free to add a little personal style and channel your inner dancer as you become more comfortable with the program.

All of the BBS programs use your own body weight and light resistance in the form of small dumbbells and bands to develop long, lean muscle tissue, so please don't worry about becoming bulky. It's a myth that strength training adds bulk. If you do it the right way, with lighter weights and more reps, you will sculpt the body of a dancer, not create the heft of a bodybuilder—I promise you! I am living proof of this.

Additional benefits of strength training include:

* improved athletic performance
* reduced risk of injury
* reduced risk of heart disease and diabetes
* increased stamina

As you progress through each workout, we will focus on different muscle groups. Some moves work the upper body, some the lower body, and some the core. Let's turn the page and look at the method behind my madness:

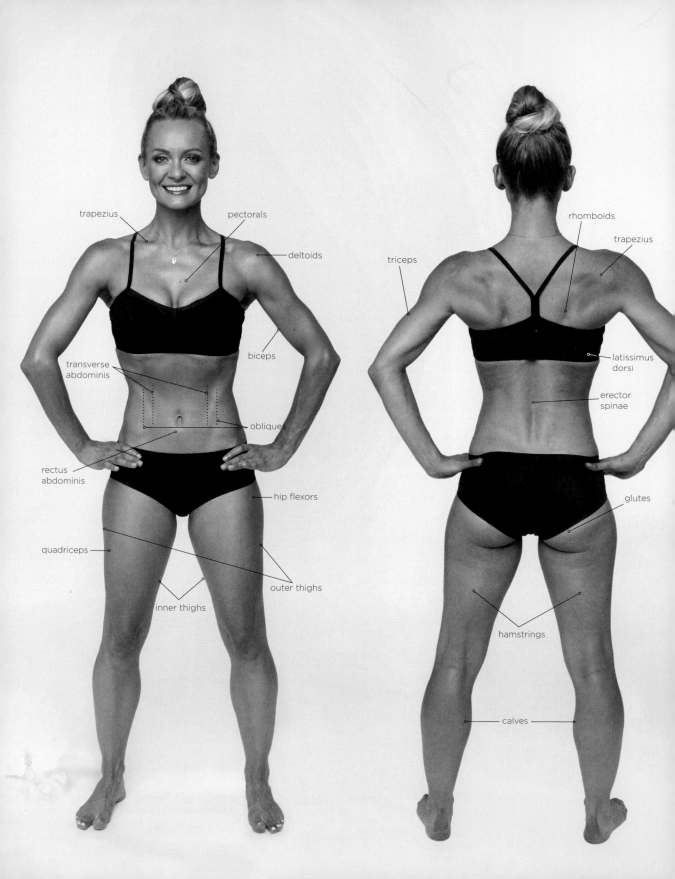

trapezius

pectorals

deltoids

biceps

transverse
abdominis

obliques

rectus
abdominis

hip flexors

quadriceps

outer thighs

inner thighs

rhomboids

trapezius

triceps

latissimus
dorsi

erector
spinae

glutes

hamstrings

calves

Upper Body

A dancer's arms are always in motion, and it's because of this perpetual movement that she develops definition in her shoulders, upper back, and chest. To augment this development, I add some small hand weights and resistance bands to help sculpt your top half quickly and efficiently.

Upper-Body Muscles Worked

- DELTOIDS: These three muscles (front, side, and rear) make up your shoulder muscle group and move your arms forward, backward, side to side, and around.
- BICEPS: This muscle runs along the front of your arm and allows you to flex (bend) your elbow.
- TRICEPS: These three muscles run along the back of your arm and work together to extend your lower arm and straighten your elbow.
- TRAPEZIUS: These muscles are located in your upper back and neck, retracting (bringing together) your shoulder blades, and supporting your arms.
- RHOMBOIDS: These muscles are located in your mid-back, supporting and holding your shoulder blades in close to your rib cage.
- LATISSIMUS DORSI: This large muscle pair runs from your shoulders and neck down to your lower back in a big triangle, allowing you to bring your arms inward and behind you, as well as to rotate them in their sockets. The "lats" also move your shoulder blades downward and inward.
- ERECTOR SPINAE: These muscles run vertically down the center of your back along your spine and allow you to stand up straight, bend side to side, and twist.
- PECTORALS: These muscles are located in your chest and allow you to rotate and raise your arms up and down, as well as raise and lower your shoulder blades.

Lower Body

Using resistance bands and a simple yoga ball, we will target your lower half to sculpt lean legs, lean hips, and a nice perky bum.

Lower-Body Muscles Worked

- QUADRICEPS: These four muscles run along the front of your thigh, extending (straightening) your knee and flexing (bending) your hip.
- HAMSTRINGS: These three muscles run along the back of your thigh from your pelvis to your knee, flexing (bending) your knee and rotating your leg inward and outward.
- GLUTES: These three muscles make up your bum (gluteus maximus, minimus, and medius) and extend (straighten) your hip, rotate your leg inward and outward, and lift your leg behind you.
- INNER THIGHS: These muscles run along the inside of your thigh from your knee to your groin and move your leg inward.
- OUTER THIGHS: These muscles run along the outside of your leg from your knee to your hip and move your leg outward.
- CALVES: These muscles are on the back of your leg between your knee and your heel and allow you to point your toes and bend your knee.

Core

Your core is the powerhouse of your whole body, and if it is strong, everything becomes easier, including ordinary daily activities. Your core muscles engage even when you do the most menial tasks, such as picking up a sack of groceries or cleaning your windows—not to mention when you exercise. A strong core is necessary to bend, lift, and twist and can compensate for a weak back. It is also essential for good posture, balance, and stability, all of which are imperative when dancing.

Core Muscles Worked

- RECTUS ABDOMINIS: This muscle—your "six-pack"—runs vertically in the center of your abdomen, from pelvis to sternum, and allows you to bend forward.

- OBLIQUES (INNER AND OUTER): These muscles run diagonally from your ribs to your pelvis and allow you to bend side to side, fold forward, and twist.
- TRANSVERSUS ABDOMINIS: This innermost abdominal muscle wraps around your midsection like a corset, supporting your spine and internal organs.
- HIP FLEXORS: This muscle group is located around each of your hip joints and works to lift your knees to the front, rotate your legs, and bring your legs inward toward your body.

Q&A

QUESTION: I already have a lot of muscle in my legs, but my arms are weaker. Can I skip the lower-body portion and do only the upper-body portion of the Strength workouts?

ANSWER: I recommend training every body part each time you exercise. Many women do a lot of cardio, which builds a strong lower body and great endurance but does little to strengthen the upper body. BBS works all your muscles from top to bottom so your upper half gets the attention it deserves. But don't worry, working your legs won't add bulky muscle, and in fact training them can help you burn more fat: since your legs contain some of the largest muscles in your body, training them can burn a ton of calories and get you that much closer to your goals! If you want to develop more muscles in your arms, use your hand weights and be sure to do each motion deliberately. Also, really work on establishing that mind-muscle connection with your upper body, feeling each rep and each muscle that you're working.

QUESTION: Isn't my "core" the same thing as my "abs"?

ANSWER: Yes and no. Your core *includes* your abs, but it also includes your hips, obliques, lower back, and glutes. Working your core is about more than just developing a six-pack. A strong core provides balance and stability for the whole body, and helps prevent lower-back strain and pain.

Level I: Corps de Ballet

STRENGTH WORKOUT

When I was at the Royal National Theatre, in London, I was in the Corps de Ballet in *A Funny Thing Happened on the Way to the Forum*. The Corps all worked together to tell the story, and not one of us was more important than the other, which is the nature of that position. Like they say, you have to start somewhere, and all ballet dancers begin in the Corps to gain some experience and discipline before they move into a Soloist or Principal position, where they can stand out. Here in Level I, you will learn the steps and build the strength and endurance to move to the next level in the BBS program.

The Nuts and Bolts

* Begin with a 5-10 minute warm-up, then start with whichever section you'd like—upper body, lower body, or core. Do all three sections each time you work out.
* True beginners should do one set of each exercise for 8-10 reps each. If you're a bit more advanced or are a few weeks into the program, shoot for 1-2 sets of 10-15 reps each. For exercises that alternate sides, complete all of the reps on one side before moving on to the other side.
* Take breaks as you need them at first, but as you get stronger, try to cut your rest time between exercises down to a minute or less. This will increase the intensity, and your calorie burn.
* After your workout, spend 5-10 minutes cooling down and stretching (see page 123).

What You'll Need

Pilates ball

towel

water

yoga mat (optional)

small dumbbells or Reebok

Thumblock wrist weights

Upper Body

Ready Position

For the next four moves, you will start in the ready position.

Stand with your feet and knees together, back straight. Bend your knees slightly and angle your torso forward with a flat back. Tighten your abs and align your head with your spine to protect your neck and upper back. With wrist weights attached or hand weights in your hands, extend your arms out behind you. Maintain this body position throughout this arm series.

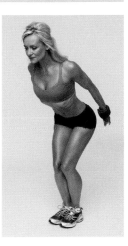

mummy modification

If you are far along in your pregnancy and it bothers you to lean forward, do these moves standing upright instead of inclined forward to avoid strain in your lower back.

TIP: This series is great if you want to tone and tighten your arms for tank-top season or to prep for that little black dress!

Swan Arms

Muscles worked: shoulders, upper back

Stand in the ready position. Extend your arms along your sides with your palms facing inward [1]. Open your arms to the side and sweep them gracefully upward, reaching out and away from your shoulders in a smooth arc until they come overhead [2]. Reverse the move and sweep them back down to complete one repetition. Do 8–15 reps.

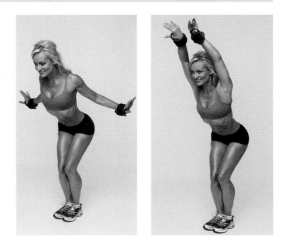

TIP: Keep your arms in the same plane as your body, extending them and reaching out and away in a large arc. This will give you a great stretch through your sides and back as well as working your shoulders.

Sliders

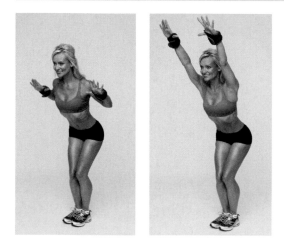

Muscles worked: shoulders, upper back, middle back

Stand in the ready position. Bend your elbows and tuck your arms in close to your sides, palms facing the floor, hands at chest level [1]. Reach upward until your arms are fully extended in line with your body, spreading your fingers and reaching for the ceiling [2]. Pull them back down to the start, squeezing your shoulder blades together on the return. Do 8–15 reps.

TIP: Press your shoulders down away from your ears as you reach overhead to lengthen and strengthen your upper back and shoulders.

Breaststroke

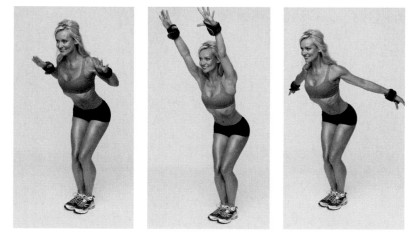

Muscles worked: shoulders, middle back, upper back

Stand in the ready position. Bend your elbows and tuck your arms in close to your sides, palms facing the floor, hands close together in front of your chest [1]. Extend your arms upward until they are straight and in line with your body [2], then open them out and circle them around and down to your sides as if taking a swimming stroke [3]. Bend your elbows and lift your hands back to the start to complete one repetition. Do 8–15 reps.

TIP: Spread your fingers and reach your arms out and away as you circle them downward.

Row and Kick

Muscles worked: middle back, triceps

Stand in the ready position. Extend your arms downward so they are perpendicular to the floor [1]. Drive your elbows up and back, keeping your arms in close to your sides and squeezing your shoulder blades together [2]. Pin your upper arms to your sides and straighten your elbows, pressing your palms toward the ceiling [3]. Reverse the move to return to the ready position. Do 8–15 reps.

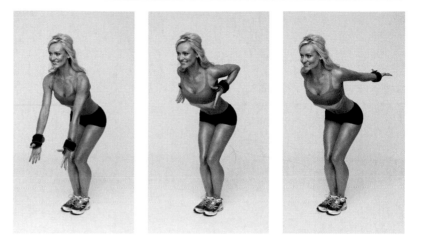

Port de Bras

Muscles worked: shoulders, upper back, chest

Stand upright with your feet wider than shoulder-width apart and extend your arms out to the sides at shoulder height [1]. Sweep your right arm up overhead, turning the palm inward and gracefully curving your arm to frame your head [2]. Continuing, circle the arm down and around, across your face and chest [3], then raise it back out to the side and up to the start to complete one repetition. Switch arms and repeat. Do 8–15 reps, each arm.

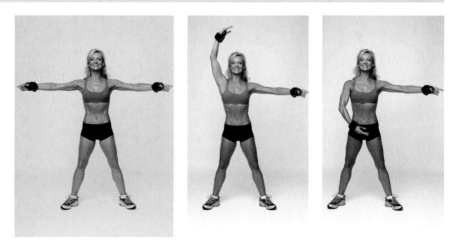

TIP: This is a great move for improving your posture. Channel your inner ballerina and make each element graceful and dramatic. Follow your hand with your gaze, turning your head to watch your hand through its trajectory.

Great Guns

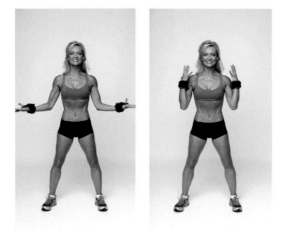

Muscles worked: biceps

Stand upright with your feet wider than shoulder-width apart, arms at your sides, and turn your palms outward [1]. Bend your elbows and bring your hands up toward your shoulders, squeezing your biceps [2]. Pause a moment at the top, then slowly lower back to the start. Do 8–15 reps.

TIP: Bring your arms slightly forward of your body and extend them fully with each repetition to work the biceps properly.

Wall Push

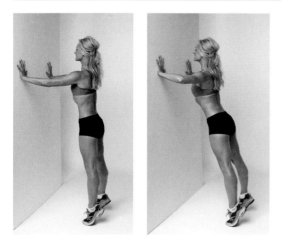

Muscles worked: chest, triceps, core

Stand facing a wall with your feet hip-width apart and your toes about 1–2 feet away from the baseboard. Place your hands flat on the wall at chest height, wider than shoulder-width apart [1]. Bend your elbows to "lower" yourself toward the wall, keeping your whole body rigid and straight [2]. When you've come as low as you comfortably can, extend your arms and push yourself away from the wall to return to the start. Do 8–15 reps.

TIP: Pretend you're a board; make sure your body stays stiff through your torso and hips as you bend and straighten your arms.

Lower Body

Tabletop Position

The starting position for the next two moves is the tabletop position.

Get on your hands and knees with your hands placed directly underneath your shoulders and your knees directly underneath your hips. Tighten your abs and flatten your back—like a table. Your head should be neutral, in line with your spine. Do this sideways to a mirror initially to make sure you're in the correct position.

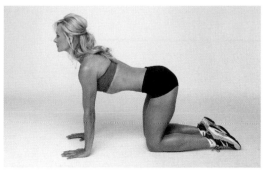

Great Glute Kick I

Muscles worked: glutes, lower back, abs

Get into the tabletop position. Extend one leg behind you in the air, parallel to the floor, with your toe pointed [1]. Bend your knee and bring your leg underneath you, tucking your knee into your chest without rounding your back [2]. Extend your leg back to the starting position to complete the repetition. Switch legs and repeat. Do 8–15 reps, each leg.

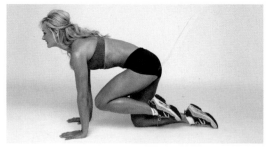

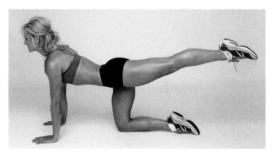

TIP: Make sure you don't wobble or lean sideways! Tighten your abs and keep your shoulders square to remain in the proper position.

Better Bun Lift I

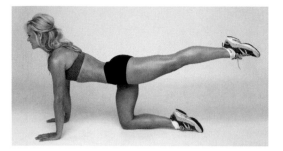

Muscles worked: glutes, lower back, hamstrings

Get into the tabletop position. Extend one leg behind you in the air so it's parallel to the floor, with your toe pointed [1]. Keeping your leg straight, lower it and tap the toe on the floor [2]. Raise it back to the starting position to complete one repetition. Do 8–15 reps, each leg.

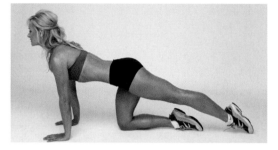

TIP: Watch yourself closely in the mirror to ensure you're not arching your back when you lift your leg into the air. And don't lift it higher than parallel to the floor!

This is a great move to lift and round out the booty!

Side Saddle

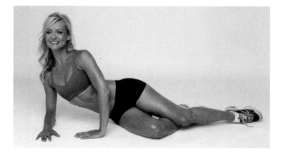

Position yourself on your side with your hips stacked. Bend your bottom leg and tuck that heel behind you. Place your bottom elbow on the floor, beneath your shoulder. Press down into this elbow to prevent sagging. Place your other hand on the floor in front of you for stability.

Side Lying

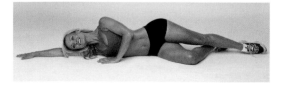

If this seated position is uncomfortable or awkward for you, you can also lie down on the floor: extend your bottom arm along the ground and rest your head on top of it. Place your top hand on the floor in front of you for balance.

For the next two moves your starting position will be a side-saddle (or side-lying) position.

Hip Slimmer I

Muscles worked: glutes, outer thighs

Get into the side-saddle position. Extend your top leg so it's straight, with your foot flexed and hovering just above the floor [1]. Raise your leg until it comes just above hip height [2], then lower back to the starting position. Roll over to your other side and repeat with the opposite leg. Do 8-15 reps, each leg.

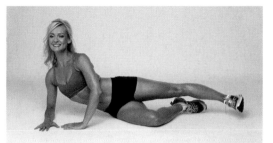

TIP: As you raise your leg, press down into your elbow to help counterbalance its weight and maintain proper form.

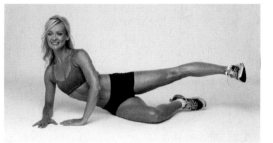

> This move is great for melting fat off of the terribly named "saddlebag" area. But you know what I mean . . .

Total Side Shaper I

Muscles worked: outer thighs, glutes, abs

Get into the side-saddle position. Extend your top leg so it's straight and parallel to the floor, with your foot flexed [1]. Bend your knee and bring it in toward your chest, keeping it parallel to the ground [2]. Extend it back to the start to complete one repetition. Roll over to your other side to repeat with the opposite leg. Do 8–15 reps, each leg.

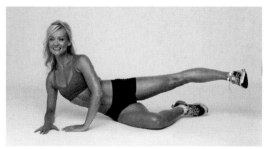

TIP: Imagine you're pressing the wall away from you as you extend back to the start, pushing through your heel and squeezing your glutes.

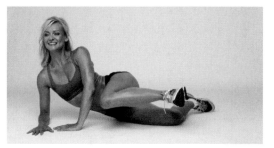

Core

C-Position

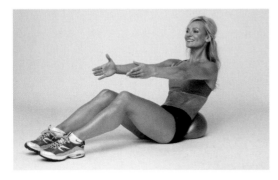

The next two moves are done in the C-position, using the Pilates ball.

Sit on the floor with your knees bent and your feet flat. Place the Pilates ball behind you in the curve of your lower back and lean against it so your torso makes a 45-degree angle to the floor. "Scoop" your abs by tucking your pelvis under slightly and creating a C-curve with your torso. Hold this position for the duration of exercises.

Pulse Crunch

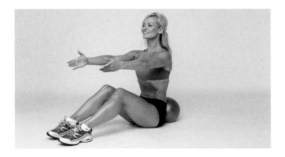

Muscles worked: abs

Get into the C-position. Extend your arms parallel to the ground and reach your hands out over your knees with your chest lifted [1]. Do small pulsing reps on the ball, sitting up a few inches, then lowering back to the start [2]. Do 8–15 reps.

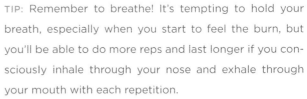

TIP: Remember to breathe! It's tempting to hold your breath, especially when you start to feel the burn, but you'll be able to do more reps and last longer if you consciously inhale through your nose and exhale through your mouth with each repetition.

mummy modification ─────

Standing Crunch: Stand with your feet hip-width apart and your fingers laced loosely behind your head. Pull your belly button in and tilt your pelvis slightly as you crunch forward, contracting your abs just as you would if you were lying on the floor. Stand back up straight to complete the rep. You can also lift one knee up in front of you as you crunch down, alternating legs with each rep. Do 8–15 reps.

Side Pulse

Muscles worked: obliques

Get into the C-position. Turn your shoulders and upper body to one side while keeping your hips square. Reach your hands to the outside of your knee and do small, pulsing reps in this position [1]. Switch sides and repeat. [2]. Do 8–15 reps, each side.

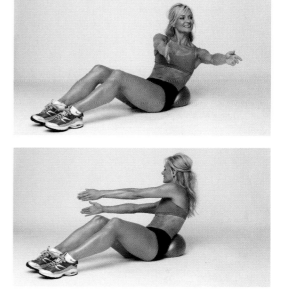

TIP: Remember to keep your chest lifted and your shoulders down away from your ears to maintain proper form!

This is the ultimate move for banishing muffin tops for good!

mummy modification

Standing Side Crunch: Stand with your feet hip-width apart, fingers laced lightly behind your head. Keeping your hips square, bend to the side, bringing your rib cage toward your hip bone, and squeeze. Stand up straight and repeat on the other side. You can also lift your knee to the side as you crunch, alternating legs with each rep. Do 8–15 reps, each side.

Plank

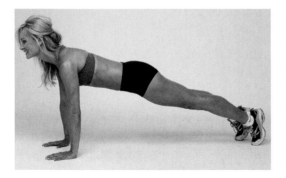

Muscles worked: abs (core), glutes, lower back, chest

Get into the tabletop position with your hands under your shoulders and your knees under your hips. Extend your legs behind you, keeping your back straight, your abs tight, and your head neutral. Hold and breathe for 20 seconds.

TIP: This is a good move to practice sideways to the mirror to ensure correct form. Your back should not sway, your hips should not rise.

The Plan

Upper Body

EXERCISE	SETS	REPS
Swan Arms	1–2	8–15
Sliders	1–2	8–15
Breaststroke	1–2	8–15
Row and Kick	1–2	8–15
Port de Bras	1–2	8–15
Great Guns	1–2	8–15
Wall Push	1–2	8–15

Lower Body

EXERCISE	SETS	REPS
Great Glute Kick I	1–2 each side	8–15
Better Bun Lift I	1–2 each side	8–15
Hip Slimmer I	1–2 each side	8–15
Total Side Shaper I	1–2 each side	8–15

Core

EXERCISE	SETS	REPS
Pulse Crunch	1–2	8–15
Side Crunch	1–2	8–15
Plank	1–2	4 (holding 20 seconds each)

Remember to drink your water! Hydration is essential when strength training, so sip it frequently throughout your workout to keep your energy level up. When you're done with your workout, polish off another glass to replenish and fuel recovery.

Level II: Soloist

STRENGTH WORKOUT

When I was in *Cats*, I was Victoria, the white cat. I had the honor of performing a three-minute solo at the beginning of the show, surrounded by darkness with only a beam of light shining down on me like the moon. This was a huge step up from the Corps de Ballet, and it was a big deal for me: it meant that I was moving ahead in my career. This Soloist workout similarly means that you have achieved your goals in Level I and are ready to challenge yourself with a more complex routine.

The Nuts and Bolts

- Start with a 5–10-minute warm-up to get ready to work out.
- Choose a section to start with—upper body, lower body, or core—then do the moves in that section in order. Do all three sections each time you work out.
- Start by going through each series one time, and as you get stronger, go through each series twice.
- You should be working in the 10–15 repetition range for each move. For

exercises that alternate sides, complete all of the reps on one side before moving on to the other side.

- Rest no more than 60 seconds between each move, and as you progress, cut the time down to 30 seconds or less.
- Rest 60 seconds between each series if needed.
- End with a 5–10-minute cool-down and stretch.

What You'll Need

small dumbbells or Reebok Thumblock Wrist Weights

Pilates ball

water

towel

Upper Body

Crisscross

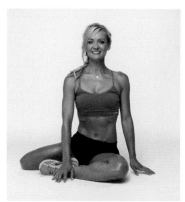

For the next seven exercises, you'll be in the crisscross position.

Sit on the floor with your left knee bent and the sole of your shoe on the inside of your right thigh. Bend your right knee and tuck the heel of your right shoe behind you and in toward your buttocks. Sit up tall with a straight spine, shoulders down, and back and head neutral. Place your left hand on the floor next to your left buttock for stability as you work your right arm. Reverse these directions to work the opposite side.

TIP: If this position is too difficult for you, or if you are pregnant and uncomfortable, try sitting cross-legged instead. Just remember to sit up tall and not to slouch!

This series really hits your shoulders and upper back, etching in definition and shape that will make you look fabulous in strapless tops and dresses!

Raise the Barre I

Muscles worked: shoulders, upper back

Sit in the crisscross position. Hold a weight at shoulder height with your arm straight in front of you, parallel to the floor [1]. Lower the weight slowly, keeping your arm straight [2], then raise it again to complete one repetition. Switch arms and repeat. Do 10–15 reps, each arm.

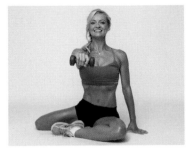

TIP: Keep your shoulders square and your neck elongated throughout this move, and focus on working your shoulder muscles.

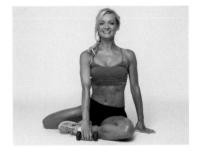

Parallel Push

Muscles worked: shoulders, upper back

Sit in the crisscross position. Hold a weight at shoulder height with one arm straight in front of you, parallel to the floor [1]. Bend your elbow and draw your arm backward, pulling your shoulder blade behind you and bringing the weight in toward your collarbone (clavicle), while keeping your arm parallel to the floor [2]. Extend back to position 1 to complete one repetition. Switch arms and repeat. Do 10–15 reps, each arm.

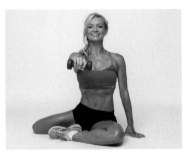

TIP: Imagine your arm is on a track, sliding in and out smoothly on the same plane as the ground.

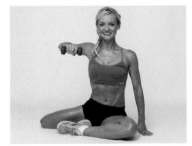

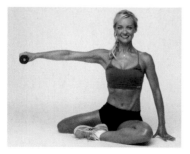

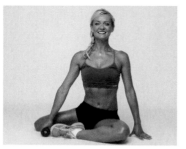

Muscles worked: shoulders, upper back

Sit in the crosscross position. Hold a weight with one arm extended to the side, parallel to the floor at shoulder height [1]. Slowly lower the weight to the floor [2], then raise it back up. Continue, using a smooth, steady motion to lift the weight up and down. Switch arms and repeat. Do 10–15 reps, each arm.

TIP: Don't lean from side to side as you raise and lower the weight; sit up tall and straight and focus on feeling the movement in your shoulder.

Stretch and Squeeze

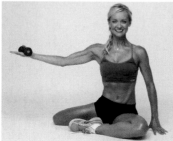

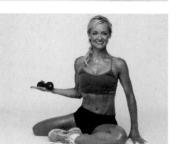

Muscles worked: shoulders, upper back, middle back

Sit in the crisscross position. Hold a weight with one arm extended to the side, parallel to the floor at shoulder height, palm facing up [1]. Bend your elbow and draw it behind you, bringing the weight in toward your shoulder and squeezing your shoulder blade behind you while keeping your arm parallel to the floor [2]. Extend back to the start to complete one repetition. Switch arms and repeat. Do 10–15 reps, each arm.

TIP: As you pull your elbow behind you, think about expanding your chest and squeezing your shoulder blades in toward your spine to get a really good contraction.

Rock and Reach

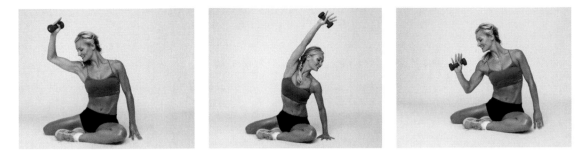

Muscles worked: shoulders, obliques

Sit in the crisscross position. Hold a weight with one arm at shoulder height with your elbow bent and tucked into your side, palm facing forward [1]. Extend your arm, reaching up first to full extension overhead, then bending over to the side, opening through your rib cage and getting a good stretch [2]. Straighten back up, then retract your arm; draw your elbow back into your side and bend the opposite way, contracting through your obliques [3]. Return to position 1 to complete one repetition. Switch arms and repeat. Do 10–15 reps, each arm.

TIP: As you reach up and over to the side, simultaneously press your opposite hip down to keep your pelvis square and increase the stretch.

Curlers

Muscles worked: biceps

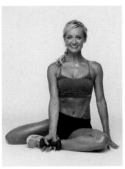
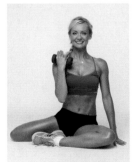

Sit in the crisscross position. Hold a weight with one arm extended down in front of you, palm facing upward [1]. Bend your elbow and curl the weight toward your shoulder, keeping your upper arm steady [2]. Reverse the move and slowly return all the way to position 1. Switch arms and repeat. Do 10–15 reps, each arm.

TIP: Make sure you bring the weight all the way back down, so your arm is straight and open to best work those beautiful biceps!

Triceps Toners

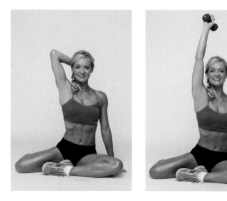

Muscles worked: triceps

Sit in the crisscross position and hold a weight in one hand. Bend forward slightly with a flat back and lift your elbow alongside your rib cage; hold your upper arm here throughout [1]. Extend your elbow, pressing the weight in a smooth arc toward the ceiling until your arm is straight [2]. Bend your elbow to return to the start, and repeat. Switch arms and repeat. Do 10–15 reps, each arm.

TIP: Make sure your shoulders are square throughout this move and that your back stays flat. Don't hunch over!

Want to eliminate arm jiggle? Curlers and Triceps Toners are your secret weapon!

Wide Pull

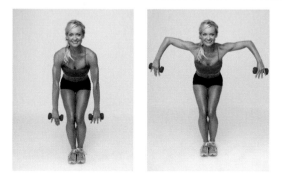

Muscles worked: middle back

Stand erect with your legs together, your knees slightly bent, and your back straight. Angle your torso forward slightly with a flat back and hold a set of dumbbells with your arms extended perpendicular to the floor, palms facing rearward [1]. Drive your elbows up and simultaneously outward, pressing the backs of your upper arms toward the ceiling. At the top, your arms should make 90-degree angles and your shoulder blades should be squeezed together, like a scarecrow [2]. Slowly lower to the start to complete one repetition. Do 10–15 reps.

TIP: Concentrate on keeping your back straight. Tighten your abs to help support the weight of your upper body and keep it flat!

Fly Away

Muscles worked: chest

Lie faceup with a weight in each hand, knees bent and feet flat on the floor. Extend your arms to the sides, palms facing upward, so your body makes a large T shape. Bend your elbows slightly and lock your arms into this position [1]. Slowly bring the weights together over your chest by raising your arms up and inward in a smooth arc until they nearly touch [2]. Slowly lower the weights back to the start to complete one repetition. Do 10–15 reps.

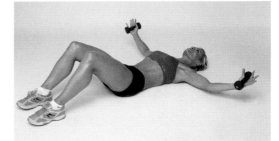

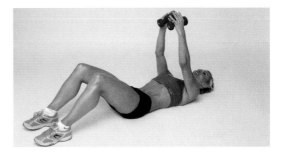

TIP: Be sure the weights come together over your chest, not your face, to work the correct muscles.

mummy modification

Lie against a medium-sized stability ball or a rolled-up yoga mat so you are at an incline to the floor and not flat on your back. Extend your arms to the sides, palms facing upward, and bend your elbows slightly, locking your arms into this position.Slowly bring the weights together over your chest by raising your arms up and inward in a smooth arc until they nearly touch. Slowly lower back to the start to complete one repetition. Do 10–15 reps.

Lower Body

For the next several exercises you'll use a soft Pilates ball and will be in either the table-top (page 65) or side-saddle/side lying (page 66) position.

Pony Kick

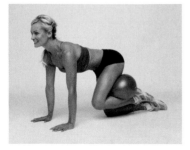

Muscles worked: glutes, hamstrings, lower back

Get into the tabletop position and place the Pilates ball in the crook of your right knee. Squeeze your heel toward your glute to secure the ball in place, foot pointed [1]. Lift your bent leg toward the ceiling until your thigh comes parallel to the floor [2]. Lower your leg to the start to complete one repetition. Switch legs and repeat. Do 10–15 reps, each leg.

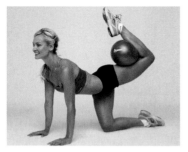

TIP: Be careful not to arch your back as you lift your leg. Keep your abs tight to support your spine and keep it neutral throughout.

Using a Pilates ball really engages the hamstrings and glutes, targeting that troublesome lower-booty area perfectly and giving your bum a lift!

Ball-abesque

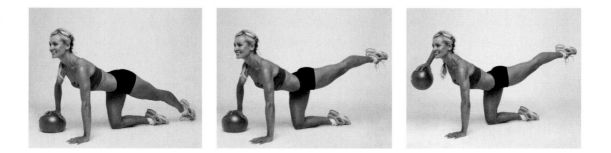

Muscles worked: glutes, lower back, shoulders, middle back

Get into the tabletop position and place the Pilates ball underneath your left hand, keeping your right hand on the floor. Extend your right leg behind you, toe pointed and just brushing the floor [1]. Raise your leg until it is parallel with the ground [2], then grip the Pilates ball with your left hand and lift it to your chest by driving your left elbow up and back [3]. Replace it on the floor and lower your leg to complete one repetition. Switch legs and repeat. Do 10–15 reps, each leg.

TIP: Keep your abs tight and your shoulders and hips square to help you maintain balance.

This exercise works your upper and lower body in the same move—it's a great time-saver!

Total Side Shaper II

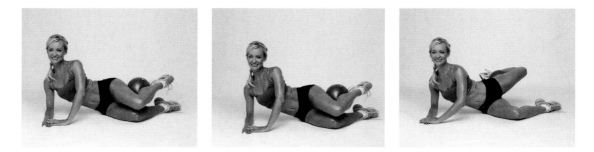

Muscles worked: glutes, outer thighs, abs

Get into the side-saddle position and squeeze the Pilates ball between the heel and glute of your top leg [1]. Bring your knee in toward your chest, keeping your leg parallel to the floor [2]. Swing your leg slowly back through the start and to the rear, squeezing your glute without arching your back [3]. Continue to move back and forth in a large arc through the air, maintaining an even pace. Roll over onto your other side and repeat with your opposite leg. Do 10–15 reps, each leg.

TIP: Keep your hips stacked throughout this move—don't lean forward or back as you move your active leg.

Glute Burnout

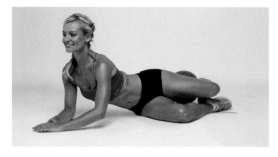

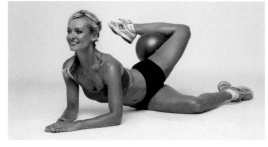

Muscles worked: glutes, outer thighs

Get into the side-saddle position and place your other forearm on the floor for balance. Squeeze the Pilates ball between the heel and the glute of your top leg [1]. Bring the leg rearward as far as you can without arching your back and hold. In this position, pulse your leg and ball up and down, slowly lifting and lowering in a short range of motion [2]. Roll over onto your other side and repeat with the opposite leg. Do 10–15 reps, each leg.

TIP: To keep from arching your back, be sure to keep your core engaged and your abs tight.

Froggy

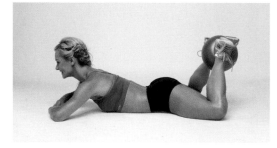

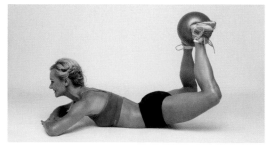

Muscles worked: glutes, lower back, hamstrings, inner thighs

Lie facedown with your legs extended behind you. Bend your knees and splay them out to the sides. Place the Pilates ball between your heels, feet flexed, and bend your knees so your shins are perpendicular to the floor and the soles of your shoes face the ceiling. Place your elbows and forearms on the floor to prop up your chest [1]. Press the soles of your shoes toward the ceiling, squeezing your glutes and lifting your knees off the floor as high as you can [2]. Lower your legs to complete one repetition. Do 10–15 reps.

TIP: The range of motion here is pretty small, so don't

force yourself to lift too high, which will compromise your form and overarch your back. Press down through your hip bones as you raise your heels toward the sky.

This is one of my favorite moves to create a nice juicy booty!

mummy modification

PLIÉ SQUAT: Stand with your feet wide, toes turned out, and place your hands on your hips. Bend your knees and squat down, tracking your knees over your toes and keeping your back straight. When your thighs come parallel to the floor, reverse the move and stand back up to the start, squeezing your bum hard at the top. Do 10–15 reps.

Leg Press I

Muscles worked: quads, hips, abs

Sit with one knee bent, foot flat on the floor, and the other leg extended in front of you, foot flexed. Lean back and rest on your elbows, keeping your abs tight and your back straight [1]. Bend the knee of your extended leg and bring it in toward your chest [2], then straighten your leg back to the start to complete one repetition. Switch legs and repeat. Do 10–15 reps, each leg.

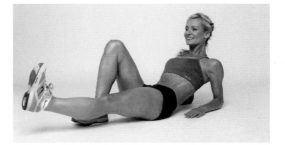

TIP: As you extend your leg at the start, imagine you're pushing the wall away from you, driving through your heel and stretching your leg away.

mummy modification

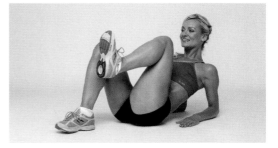

CHAIR SQUAT: Stand in front of a chair with your feet hip-width apart, hands on your hips. Squat down, bending your knees and kicking your hips back until your bum lightly touches the seat of the chair. Reverse the move, extending your legs and standing back up to the start. Do 10–15 reps.

NOTE: If you are further along in your pregnancy, stand with your feet a little wider and turned out slightly, and use a taller chair.

Core

Roll Ups

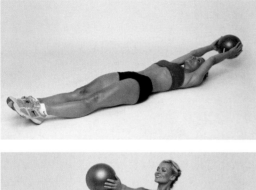

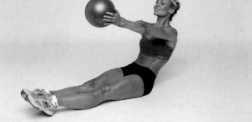

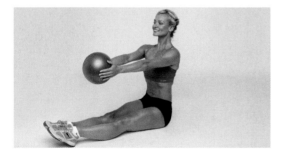

Muscles worked: abs, hips

Hold the Pilates ball in both hands and lie faceup with your legs together. Reach your arms overhead so the ball hovers just above the floor [1]. Keeping your arms straight, sweep the ball overhead smoothly and curl up, leading with your head and neck [2], then your shoulders, and finally your back and torso. At the top you should be sitting up tall, back straight, arms parallel to the floor, legs straight [3]. Roll back slowly, placing one vertebra at a time on the floor until you return to the start to complete one rep. Do 10 reps.

TIP: You may be tempted to use the weight of your legs to "kick" up and help you rise. Avoid this by consciously driving your heels into the ground as you sit up to force your core to work harder.

mummy modification

Seated crunch: Sit with one knee bent, foot flat on the floor, and the other leg extended straight in front of you. Place your hands behind you with your fingertips facing your glutes, and lift your chest. Bend the knee of your extended leg and bring it in toward your chest, simultaneously crunching forward gently. Extend your leg back along the ground and lean back slightly. Switch legs and repeat. Do 10 reps each side.

Plank

The next two moves are done in plank position.

Get into the tabletop position, your hands under your shoulders and your knees under your hips. Extend your legs behind you, keeping your back straight, your abs tight, and your head neutral.

Single Knee Drops

Muscles worked: abs (core), lower back, obliques, glutes, hamstrings, chest

Get into the plank position [1]. Without lifting your toes, bend one knee and touch it to the floor. Keep your body solid and straight [2]! Straighten your leg and squeeze your glute to return to position 1. Switch legs and repeat. Do 5 reps, each leg.

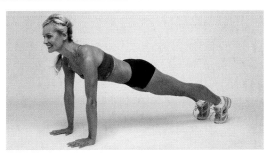

TIP: Don't lean to the side or allow your hips to rise or sag! The only thing that should be moving is your knee, bending and straightening.

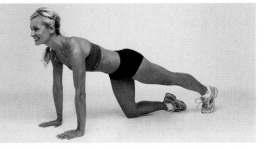

Talk about a multitasking move: this works the abs, back, arms, chest, glutes, and hamstrings all at once!

Single Towel Slider

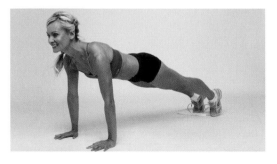

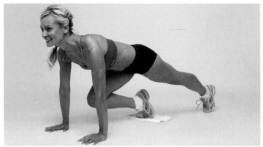

Muscles worked: abs (core), lower back, glutes, chest, hamstrings

Get into the plank position and place a small hand towel underneath your toes [1]. Bend your knee and draw it underneath you in toward your chest, sliding the towel along the floor [2]. Extend your leg back to position 1 to complete one repetition. Switch legs and repeat. Do 5–10 reps, each leg.

NOTE: If you're working on carpet, use a paper plate instead of a towel!

Keep your hips low as you draw your knee underneath you; don't round or arch your back.

The Plan

Upper Body

EXERCISE	SETS	REPS
Raise the Barre I	1–2	10–15
Parallel Push	1–2	10–15
Single Shoulder Shaper	1–2	10–15
Stretch and Squeeze	1–2	10–15
Rock and Reach	1–2	10–15
Curlers	1–2	10–15
Triceps Toners	1–2	10–15
Wide Pull	1–2	10–15
Fly Away	1–2	10–15

Lower Body

EXERCISE	SETS	REPS
Pony Kick	1–2	10–15
Ball-abesque	1–2	10–15
Total Side Shaper II	1–2	10–15
Glute Burnout	1–2	10–15
Froggy	1–2	10–15
Leg Press I	1–2	10–15

Core

EXERCISE	SETS	REPS
Roll Ups	1–2	10
Single Knee Drops	1–2	5 each leg
Single Towel Sliders	1–2	5–10 each leg

Level III: Principal

STRENGTH WORKOUTS

I performed in the musical *Fame* as Iris the ballet dancer. It was my very first Principal role and I was thrilled to have finally achieved a lifelong dream. I was also delighted to be able to combine my classical ballet training with my musical-theater experience, putting it all together and becoming a well-rounded performer. In Level III, you'll get to combine what you've learned in the Corps de Ballet and Soloist training to become a Principal in your own right.

The Nuts and Bolts

- Begin with a 5–10-minute warm-up to prepare your body to work out.
- Choose a series to start with, then do all the moves, in order, with little to no rest in between. Do all three series each time you exercise.
- Go through each series 2–3 times, resting no more than 60 seconds between rounds. For exercises that alternate sides, complete all of the reps on one side before moving on to the other side.

- Do the suggested number of reps for each move. Once this gets easy, it's time to get a "heavier" band, or increase the tension on your band by making it shorter.
- Finish with a 5–10-minute cool-down and stretch.

What You'll Need

resistance bands
Pilates ball

water
towel

A Note on Resistance Bands

When using a resistance band, stand with your feet shoulder-width apart on the center of the band and grip the handles tightly. If you're using a band without handles, wrap the ends securely several times around your hands so they do not come loose.

The nature of a rubber band when stretched is to snap back to its natural position. Therefore, the more you pull it out of shape, the greater it will resist your pull. The key with bands is to maintain that resistance throughout the exercise. At no point do you want to give in to the band and let it snap back into place! You control its tension and motion with your muscles. You make it stretch, then allow it to *slowly* return to normal. This is the most effective way to do the exercises, as it creates the most tension and the most work. It also keeps you from getting snapped by the band!

If you don't have a band, you can use dumbbells for this series as well.

Upper Body

For these moves you'll be in an "athletic" position.
Stand with your feet hip-width apart, your knees slightly bent and your shoulders down and back. Pull your abs in tight and keep your head neutral.

86

Band Curlers

Muscles worked: biceps

Get into the athletic position and hold a band end in each hand with your palms turned outward [1]. Bend your elbows, curling your hands toward your shoulders while keeping your elbows in close to your body [2]. Lower your arms slowly, resisting the pull of the band on the return to the starting position. Do 15–20 reps.

TIP: Maintain good posture—keep your shoulders down and your back straight. Use your core to keep you steady, and feel the burn in your biceps.

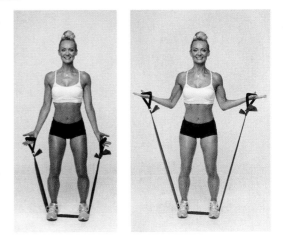

Double Curl and Reach

Muscles worked: biceps, shoulders, upper back

Get into the athletic position and hold a band end in each hand, palms turned outward [1]. Bend your elbows to curl both hands toward your shoulders, squeezing the biceps [2]. Then press both hands up overhead and turn your wrists so your palms face front at the top [3]. Reverse the move to return to position 1. Do 15–20 reps.

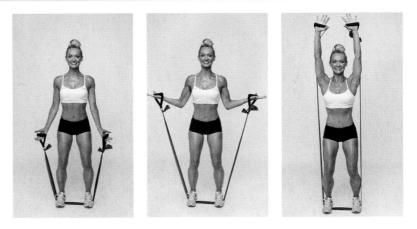

TIP: Make sure you're using a lighter band for this move—pressing it overhead should be challenging but not impossible!

This is a great way to sculpt sexy arms—you hit your biceps and shoulders at the same time.

87

Airplane

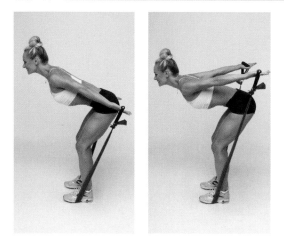

Muscles worked: triceps, middle back, lower back

Stand in the athletic position and hold a band end in each hand. Fold your torso forward with a flat back about 45 degrees and extend your arms along your sides, palms facing the sky [1]. Press your arms up toward the ceiling, keeping your torso steady and your back flat [2]. Lower arms to position 1 and repeat. Do 15–20 reps.

TIP: Don't bend your elbows; keep your arms as straight as possible throughout.

Double Shoulder Shaper

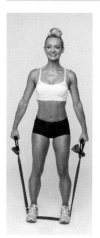
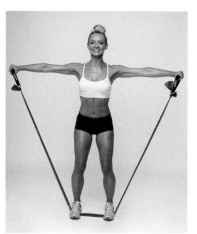

Muscles worked: shoulders, upper back

Get into the athletic position and hold a band end in each hand, palms facing inward [1]. Lift both arms smoothly up and out to the sides, raising them to shoulder height, parallel to the floor. At the top you should resemble a T-shape. [2]. Slowly lower your arms to the starting position, resisting the pull of the band on the return. Do 15–20 reps.

TIP: To maintain proper position, think about leading this motion with your elbows, not your hands.

Double Raise the Barre

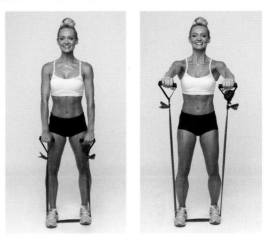

Muscles worked: shoulders, upper back

Stand with your arms extended in front of your thighs, holding a band end in each hand, with your palms facing your legs [1]. Keeping your arms straight, raise them up in front of you to shoulder height [2]. Pause briefly, then slowly lower to the start, resisting the pull of the band on the return. Do 15–20 reps.

TIP: You may have a tendency to lean back as you lift the band—resist this temptation! Stand up tall and make your shoulders do all the work. If you feel like you *have* to lean back, you might need to switch to a lighter band.

Anchors Aweigh: How to Secure Your Band

A few of the exercises in this book will require you to "anchor" your band with something other than your feet, so that when you pull the band it is parallel to the floor rather than perpendicular. Most resistance-band kits come with an anchor, a loop of nylon with a ball on the end that you can shut into a door, securing the band and enabling you to use it from different angles. If you don't have an anchor, loop the center of the band on the outside doorknob then close the door tightly to secure the band in place. You can also loop the band around a heavy piece of furniture, such as a bedpost. When a move requires an anchor, I have notated it with the word "ANCHOR."

One-Arm Pull and Twist (ANCHOR)

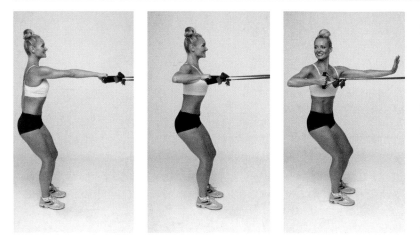

Muscles worked: middle back, obliques

Anchor a band at shoulder height and take both ends in your right hand. Face the anchor, then take a large step away to create tension in the band. Extend your arm straight out from your shoulder, parallel to the floor [1]. Pull the band toward your chest by driving your right elbow back and squeezing your shoulder blade behind you [2]. Hold here and turn your shoulders to the right, twisting your waist as you turn [3]. Return to position 1 to complete one repetition. Switch arms and repeat. Do 15–20 reps, each side.

TIP: As you perform the twist, take a deep inhale and exhale forcefully, then twist a little farther, if you can.

The pull-and-twist motion of this exercise really helps tighten the muscles in your waist and hips.

Chest Fly (ANCHOR)

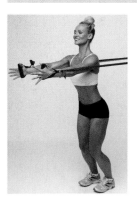
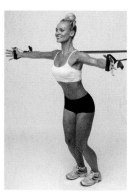

Muscles worked: chest, shoulders

Anchor the band at chest height and take an end in each hand. Turn away from the anchor so that it is behind you and step forward to create tension in the band. Extend your arms in front of you at chest height, palms facing inward, elbows slightly bent [1]. Open your arms out to the side, keeping a slight bend in the elbows [2]. Do 15–20 reps, each arm.

TIP: Don't open your arms too wide in this move—stop when your elbows come even with your rib cage.

Lower Body

You may want to use a yoga mat for these moves to provide a bit of cushioning from the floor.

Great Glute Kick II

Muscles worked: glutes, hamstrings, abs

Get into tabletop position and loop the center of the band across the sole of your right shoe, foot flexed. Hold a band end in each hand and lift your right leg off the floor an inch or so [1]. Draw your right knee underneath you into your chest, keeping your back flat and your hips square [2]. Extend your right leg away from you, pressing against the band and straightening your leg until it's parallel to the floor [3]. Continue with an even cadence for all your reps. Switch legs and repeat. Do 15–20 reps, each leg.

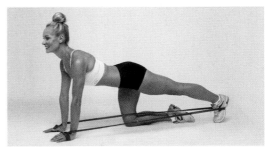

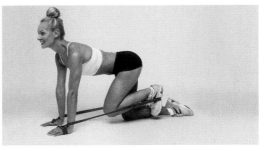

TIP: Keeping your foot flexed and moving your leg in a straight trajectory will help keep the band from slipping. This exercise is much easier to do with sneakers on, so if you've taken them off for any reason, be sure to put them back on.

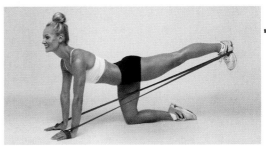

You don't have to use the same band for every exercise. For exercises that feel easy to you, use a "heavier" band. If a move proves especially challenging, switch to a "lighter" band and stick with it until you're able to do all of the reps with proper form.

You can also increase the tension of a band by shortening the length you hold, or decrease the tension by creating more slack, or length, in the band.

Better Bun Lift II

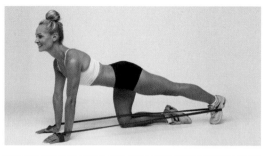

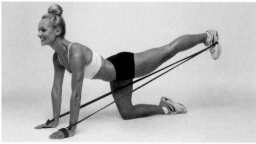

Muscles worked: glutes, hamstrings

Get into the tabletop position and hold a band end in each hand. Loop the center of the band across the sole of your right shoe, foot flexed, and extend your right leg away from you, toe touching the ground [1]. Lift your leg until it's parallel to the floor [2], then lower to position 1. Switch legs and repeat. Do 15-20 reps, each leg.

TIP: The tension in the band will make you want to bend your knee—fight back! Press your heel away from you to further engage your hamstrings and glutes.

Hip Slimmer II

Muscles worked: glutes, outer thighs, abs

Get into the side-saddle position and loop the center of the band around the instep of your top shoe, foot flexed. Hold both ends of the band in front of you on the floor. Bend your knee and bring it into your chest [1]. Extend your leg away from you, parallel to the floor, pressing against the band until it's straight [2]. Bring your knee back in to your chest and return to position 1 to complete one repetition. Roll onto your other side, switch legs, and repeat. Do 15–20 reps, each leg.

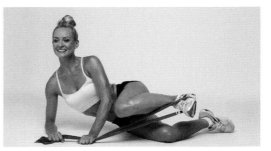

TIP: Remember to keep your hips stacked as you move your leg in and out. You should really feel your hips burning—that's fat melting away from the "saddlebag" region. Power through that burn!

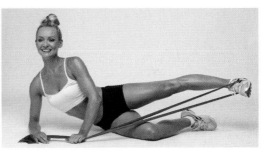

Leg Press II

Muscles worked: quads, hamstrings, glutes

Lie faceup with your left knee bent, foot flat on the floor. Loop the center of the band around the instep of your right shoe and hold an end in each hand at your sides. Extend your right leg until it's straight [1], then bend your knee and bring it in toward your abdomen [2]. Extend to position 1 to complete one rep. Do 15–20 reps, each leg.

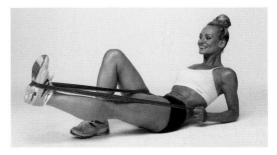

TIP: Move your leg smoothly in and out and engage your core to keep your body from tilting to the other side while you extend your leg.

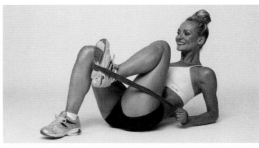

Thigh High

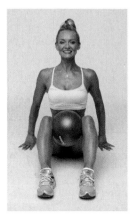 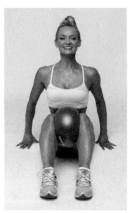

Muscles worked: inner thighs

Sit with your knees bent, feet flat, and place the Pilates ball between your knees. Place your hands on the floor behind your hips for stability and lift your chest so your back is straight [1]. Alternately squeeze and release the ball between your knees, using a steady, even motion [2]. Do 15–20 reps.

TIP: Sit up tall with your shoulders down and your back straight throughout this exercise. The range of motion is small, so make sure you fully release after each rep to maximize muscle burn.

Marching Band

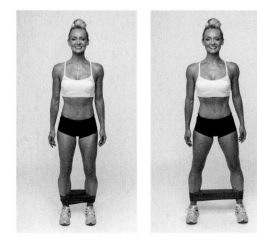

Muscles worked: outer thighs

Tie the ends of your resistance band together so that it makes a secure circle (like a giant rubber band) and loop it twice around your legs. Secure it around either your mid-thigh (easier) or your ankles (harder) and stand with your feet about hip-width apart, just far enough to create tension in the band so it stays in place [1]. Step laterally to the right and to the left, keeping your legs straight and maintaining tension in the band [2]. Do 15–20 reps.

TIP: If you have more than one band at home, it's helpful to keep one tied in a loop at the right resistance for exercises like this. Otherwise you will need to tie and untie the band each time you use it.

Core

Roll Up and Twist

Muscles worked: abs, obliques, hip flexors

Sit up tall with your back straight and your legs extended in front of you. Hold a Pilates ball in front of you, straight out from your chest, arms parallel to the floor [1]. Twist your shoulders, hands, and ball to one side while keeping your back straight [2]. Slowly roll down to the floor while still reaching to the side, lowering your back, shoulders, and then your head. Lower the ball behind your head with straight arms [3], then reverse the move, raising the arms and curling back up to return to position 1. Twist to the other side and repeat. Continue, alternating sides. Do 15–20 reps, each side.

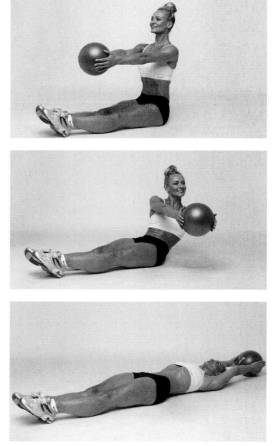

TIP: Do this move very slowly to prevent yourself from relying on momentum to complete it. Try to press your hips and glutes down into the floor to stay grounded and centered as you move from side to side; both hips should stay on the floor at all times.

mummy modification ————————

MARIONETTE: Stand with your feet hip-width apart, fingers laced loosely behind your head. Lift one knee up and out to the side, bringing that same-side elbow down toward your knee, bending to the side and squeezing your obliques. Bring your foot back down and return to the starting position. Continue, alternating sides. Do 15–20 reps, each side.

Core: Plank Series

The next five moves are done in plank position. Get into the tabletop position, your hands under your shoulders and your knees under your hips. Extend your legs behind you, keeping your back straight, your abs tight, and your head neutral.

Great Glute Kick III

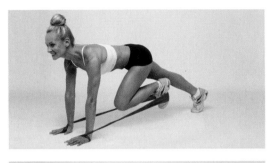

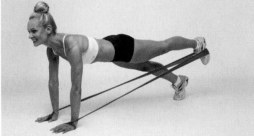

Muscles worked: abs, glutes, chest

In a sitting position, loop the center of a band around the instep of one shoe, foot flexed, and hold a band end in each hand. Get into plank position. Bend your banded leg and bring your knee underneath you and into your chest [1]. Extend it away from you, pressing against the band while keeping your hips square [2]. Do 15–20 reps, each leg.

TIP: As you extend your leg behind you, remember not to arch your back. Keep your core engaged to protect your spine.

Better Bun Lift III

Muscles worked: glutes, hamstrings, chest, abs

In a sitting position, loop the center of a band around the instep of one shoe, foot flexed, and hold a band end in each hand. Get into plank position. Extend your banded leg behind you parallel to the floor [1]. Lower your leg until your toe touches the floor [2], then raise it back up to complete one repetition. Do 15–20 reps, each leg.

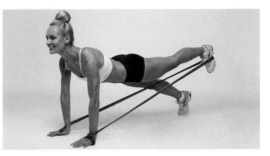

TIP: Root yourself to the floor and prevent tilting by spreading out your fingers and pressing them into the floor to distribute your body weight and help you stay square.

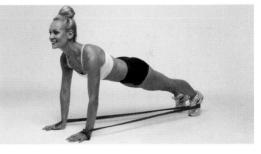

Double Knee Drops

Muscles worked: abs, chest, glutes, hamstrings

Get into plank position [1]. Bend both knees and touch them briefly to the floor [2]. Straighten your legs again to complete one rep. Do 10 reps.

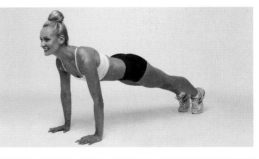

TIP: This exercise is deceptively simple! Engage your core and keep your hips lifted to maintain proper position. Your legs should be the only part of you moving.

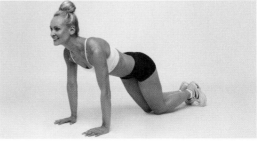

Double Towel Slider

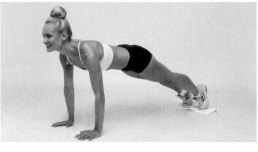

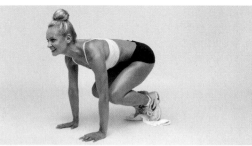

Muscles worked: abs, glutes, chest

Get into plank position and place toes of both feet on a hand towel [1]. Bend both knees and bring them underneath your body and into your chest [B]. Slowly extend your legs back to the start, keeping your core tight to maintain control. Do 10 reps.

TIP: Make sure your back does not round as you bring your knees in, and that your hips stay low. If you're working on carpet, use a paper plate instead of a towel.

Window Washer

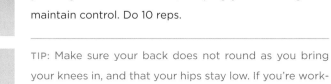

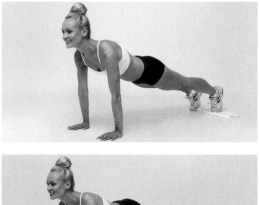

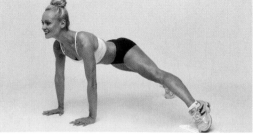

Muscles worked: abs, chest, glutes, outer thighs, inner thighs

Get into plank position and place a hand towel underneath the toes of one foot [1]. Open one leg out to the side, dragging the towel in a large arc along the floor as wide as you can go [2]. Bring your leg back in and drag the towel back to meet your other foot to complete one rep. Do 5–10 reps, each leg.

TIP: Everyone will have a different range of motion with this exercise. Extend your leg as far to the side as you can, and each time you extend, try to create a wider arc. Being consistent with your flexibility training will really help you increase your range of motion—you will notice your progress when you do this exercise.

This is one of the very best moves to hit your entire body from head to toe! There's hardly a muscle that is not working with this one.

The Plan

Upper Body

EXERCISE	SETS	REPS
Band Curlers	2–3	15–20
Double Curl and Reach	2–3	15–20
Airplane	2–3	15–20
Double Shoulder Shaper	2–3	15–20
Double Raise the Barre	2–3	15–20
One-arm Pull and Twist	2–3 each side	15–20
Chest Fly	2–3 each side	15–20

Lower Body

Remember to do both sides!

EXERCISE	SETS	REPS
Great Glute Kick II	2–3	15–20
Better Bun Lift II	2–3	15–20
Hip Slimmer II	2–3	15–20
Leg Press II	2–3	15–20
Thigh High	2–3	15–20
Marching Band	2–3	15–20

Core

EXERCISE	SETS	REPS
Great Glute Kick III	2–3	15–20
Better Bun Lift III	2–3	15–20
Double Knee Drops	2–3	10
Double Towel Slider	2–3	10
Window Washer	2–3	5–10

Chapter 8
Working Up a Sweat

And those who were seen dancing were thought to be insane by those who could not hear the music.

—FRIEDRICH NIETZSCHE

When most people think of cardio they imagine themselves plodding along on a treadmill for hours, going nowhere. Personally, I'd rather turn up the music and dance around a room than run in place! Cardiovascular exercise blasts fat and helps you build a strong heart and lungs. It also offers a host of other health benefits:

- BLUES BUSTER: Women who get 30–60 minutes of cardiovascular exercise 3–5 times per week are less likely to be depressed than women who don't exercise regularly.
- BRAIN BOOSTER: Because it increases circulation, delivering more blood, oxygen, and nutrients to the brain, doing cardiovascular exercise on a workday can boost productivity by 23%!

- HORMONE HELPER: Cardio activity causes your muscles to send hormones and chemicals to the brain that enhance memory, problem solving, and decision making. It also promotes the release of serotonin (a mood enhancer), dopamine (which affects attention and learning), and norepinephrine (which affects attention, perception, motivation, and arousal).
- DISEASE DESTROYER: Doing regular aerobic exercise can reduce your risk of breast cancer by 20–40%, and reduce your risk of colon cancer by 30–40%! It also reduces your chance of developing diabetes by more than half.

With all of this in mind, I've created three unique cardio routines that combine dance, strength training, and good old-fashioned fun so your cardio sessions will be anything but boring. Once you get the basic choreography down, trust me, you're going to have a good time with this. So let's get moving, get sweaty, and get sexy.

The Routines

Just like the strength-training workouts, my cardio routines are broken up into three different fitness levels. And while they are dance-based, don't worry—you don't have to be a dancer to do them properly. Every routine is broken down into its most basic components. I suggest practicing each move a few times before putting on your music and going for it. Some moves will become second nature in a minute and others might take a little practice, but remember—no one is watching. Dancing is about fun and exuberance; let yourself go and work up a sweat!

I've also created a jump-rope routine for each level for variety as well as those days when you're just not in the mood to dance. Jumping rope is an awesome cardio workout—it can burn up to 600 calories an hour! Another great thing about the jump-rope routines is that you can do them anywhere. And jump ropes are lightweight and portable, so you don't have an excuse to skip your workout when you're on the road!

Jump to It

If you're like most people, you probably haven't picked up a jump rope since you were a kid. No worries—you can jump like a pro with these pointers:

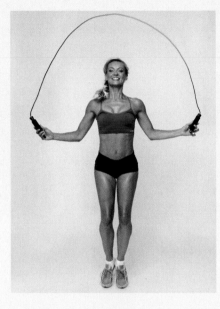

- Make sure your rope is the right length. Stand in its center and hold the ends; the handles should come to your sternum when pulled taut.
- Keep your shoulders down and your arms comfortably bent, elbows about a foot away from your sides at waist level.
- Turn the rope with your wrists and forearms, not your whole arm.
- Jump just a few inches up and down, landing on the balls of your feet. The rope is only about a quarter of an inch thick—no need to leap a foot in the air! You'll wear yourself out quickly if you're jumping too high.
- Start slowly and establish a good rhythm.
- If you have problems with your knees or hips, consider jumping on a padded surface to cushion your joints.
- Wear shoes with soles that can help absorb the shock (like running shoes), and a snug sports bra!

Counting Music

Anyone who has danced before is probably familiar with counting the beats in music. But if you haven't, don't worry—it's not hard. Here's all you need to know: most songs you'll hear on the radio are in 4:4 time, meaning there are 8 counts with each "phrase" of music. With this in mind, I use multiples of 4 and 8 when charting out the routines so they will work for your playlist. Of course, you can completely ignore this counting business if you'd like and do 10 or 20 or as many reps of each move if that suits you. As long as you're moving and your heart rate is elevated and you're having fun, you'll be just fine!

Mirror Minutes

Because dancing is so personal and intimate, I suggest doing your Mirror Minutes before doing your cardio routine, even if you've just done them before your strength training. These cardio workouts are a whole different animal, and you'll be moving in a different way and connecting with yourself in a different manner, so you may find it helpful to shift gears into dance mode by doing this exercise again.

So go ahead—give yourself a good eyeballing in the mirror. Smile at yourself, admire your shape and your body, maybe even give yourself a compliment out loud. Take five deep breaths to clear your head and shake out your limbs. Get loose and limber and liquid, then press play. You're ready to rock!

Cardio and Yummy Mummies

Cardio is great for pregnant women as well as new moms. It helps burn calories and, contrary to what you might think, gives you a boost of energy—something you really need when you're sleep deprived! If you're pregnant, remember to listen to your body—if you're too hot or tired to continue exercising, stop and take a break. Postpartum moms should start with the Level I: Corps de Ballet Cardio Workouts, and move up from there. And dance where your baby can see you! Put him or her in the bouncy seat or bassinet and do your workout where they can watch.

Cardio Warm-Up

If you've just completed your strength workout, that is sufficient as a warm-up for your cardio and you don't need to do anything extra. But if you're doing your cardio workout first as I recommend, spend 5–10 minutes warming up. Put on a song and start moving (see page 39 for some warm-up ideas). Just be sure to make it low impact—no jumping, hopping, or leaping yet. Make sure you're completely warm and limber before you start to ratchet it up. You might even want to ease into the routine by choosing a less up-tempo song for the first workout and modifying the dance moves to be low impact.

Q&A

QUESTION: I did my cardio workout yesterday and was gasping for air in the first few minutes. What gives?

ANSWER: It could be a few things. First, your music might be too fast. Try a slower selection of songs and see if that helps. You might also be working in a level that is a little too advanced for you. Try the next level down and see if that suits your ability better.

QUESTION: I want to try the jump-rope routine, but I step on the rope all the time. How do I get better at this?

ANSWER: Practice, practice, practice! Everyone steps on the rope a lot when they first begin, but you'll get better more quickly than you think. Read through the jump-rope pointers on page 102 and make any adjustments necessary. And keep at it: when you step on the rope, get right back into position and try again.

QUESTION: What are the best shoes to wear for my cardio?

ANSWER: I recommend shoes with good support that are not too rigid. Cross trainers, dance shoes, and even lightweight running shoes (I love Newtons, personally) will work for your cardio workouts.

Look For: Low-Impact Tips

Got problematic knees? Unhappy hips? Then make any move low impact by taking out the jumping, hopping, and bouncing and keep one foot on the ground at all times. I've offered Low-Impact Tips throughout the cardio workouts for more complicated moves. Doing the low-impact version of a move is also a great way to learn it before you start to rock it out.

Level I: Corps de Ballet

CARDIO WORKOUT

As a member of the Corps de Ballet in a performance, you are expected to be methodical, precise, and exact. That's just how I recommend approaching your cardio workout. Do each move with deliberate intent, and maintain a moderate pace. You're building a solid foundation from which to leap when it's time to step up to Soloist!

Jump Rope 1

Time: 5 minutes

Jumping rope takes patience and practice. Just start slowly and stick with it. If you can't jump rope for the full five minutes, jump as long as you can, march or jog in place until you recover, then begin jumping again. As the days and weeks go by, work toward building up your endurance until you can do five minutes without stopping.

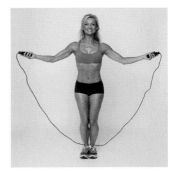

BASIC JUMP: Jump with both feet together. Remember to land lightly on the balls of your feet and don't jump too high. Play with your tempo and rhythm and have fun!

Get-on-the-Ball Routine

Time: 10 minutes

This is a fun, easy-to-learn routine that uses the Pilates ball in creative ways. Start by doing this workout for ten minutes and work up to 15 or 20 minutes as the weeks progress. Remember to take breaks when you need them, and to sip water frequently to stay hydrated. Lose yourself in the music and the time will fly by!

What You'll Need

Pilates ball

water

towel

The Plan

Make sure you have plenty of space to move around and put on your Cardio playlist.

This routine will last about 2–4 songs, depending on how long they are. That should come out to about 10 minutes total. Each week, try to add another song, and change up your playlist to keep it fresh.

If you need to take a short break, that's fine, but be sure you keep moving! If you stop moving cold turkey your muscles will cool down and could cramp or feel tight when you start again.

THE MOVE	THE REPS	THE MUSICAL COUNT
Can-can	4 to the right	8
Can-can	4 to the left	8
Riverdance	4 to the right	8
Riverdance	4 to the left	8
Ball Jack	4	8
Jack Press	4	8
Lo-Jack	4	8
The Twist	8	8

Can-can

Stand with your feet together and hold the Pilates ball with both hands directly overhead. Jump your feet apart into a split stance, with one foot forward, the other foot back [1]. Hop and bring your knee forward, simultaneously bringing the ball down to meet your knee [2]. Hop and return to the split stance, raising the ball back overhead. Do 4 reps (8 counts), each side.

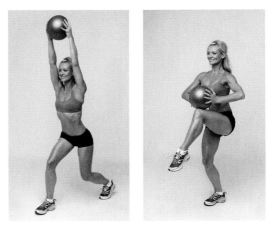

Riverdance

Face forward and reach with the Pilates ball diagonally overhead to the left. Extend your right leg out to the side, toe touching the floor [1]. Hop and bend your right knee, bringing your heel up in front of you and opening your leg to the side. Simultaneously bring your arms across your body and touch the ball with your right heel [2]. Hop and return to position 1. Switch legs and repeat. Do 4 reps, each side (8 counts).

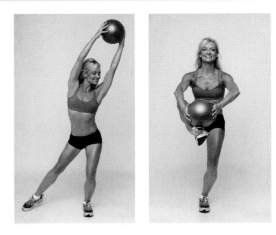

Ball Jack

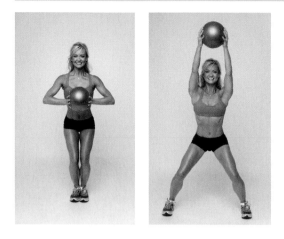

Stand with your feet and knees together and hold the Pilates ball with both hands in front of your chest, elbows bent [1]. Jump your legs apart and open and press the ball straight up overhead [2]. Jump your legs back together and bring your arms down to the start position to complete one rep. Do 4 reps, each side (8 counts).

LOW-IMPACT TIP: As you reach your arms overhead, extend one leg to the side and tap your toe on the floor. Continue, alternating sides.

Jack Press

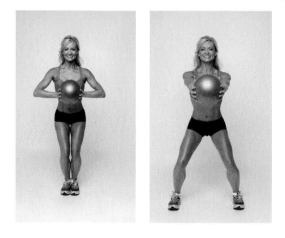

Stand with your feet and knees together and slightly bent, and hold the Pilates ball with both hands in front of your chest, elbows bent [1]. Jump your legs apart and open, and press the ball straight forward, so your arms are parallel to the floor at full extension [2]. Jump your legs back together and retract your arms to return to position 1. Do 4 reps (8 counts).

LOW-IMPACT TIP: As you press the ball forward, reach back and tap one toe to the rear. Continue, alternating legs. Do 4 reps (8 counts).

Lo-Jack

Stand with your feet and knees together and hold the ball with both hands at your chest, elbows bent [1]. Jump your feet apart and open, and reach the ball to the floor, bending forward slightly with a flat back to touch it to the ground [2]. Jump your feet back together and stand back up, returning to position 1. Do 4 reps (8 counts).

LOW-IMPACT TIP: Stand with your feet wide and hold the ball in front of your chest. Bend both knees and squat down as you reach the ball to the floor, keeping your back flat and your chest lifted. Straighten your knees and lift the ball back up to complete one rep. Do 4 reps (8 counts).

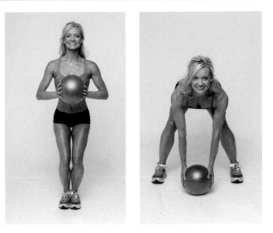

The Twist

Stand with your feet and legs together and hold the ball out in front of your chest with straight arms, parallel to the floor. Jump and twist your hips to the left while twisting your arms to the right [1]. Jump and switch, bringing hips to the right and arms and ball to the left [2]. Continue, alternating sides each time. Do 8 reps (8 counts).

LOW-IMPACT TIP: Twist and reach the ball side to side as you alternately tap your heels side to side. Do 8 reps (8 counts).

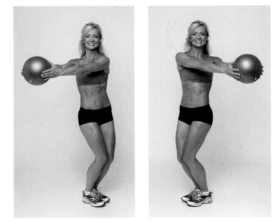

Level II: Soloist

CARDIO WORKOUT

As a dance Soloist, the show's director expects you to step up your game and stand out from the crowd, and I expect the same from you! It's time to push yourself and give your Cardio Workouts as much energy as you can. Explore your limits. You can always do a little more than you think you can!

Jump Rope II

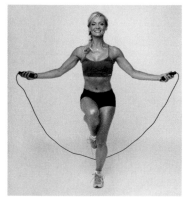

Time: 10 minutes

If you've become comfortable with the jump rope, try challenging yourself with the footwork options below. You can also increase the intensity of your jump rope routine by simply jumping faster!

REMEMBER: If you need to take a break, don't just stop—keep moving to ensure that your muscles stay warm.

footwork options

SINGLE-LEGGED HOPS: Jump rope on one foot for several revolutions, then switch feet. Remember, you only need to hop a few inches to clear the rope. Keeping your jumps low will save your energy, and your ankles!

TWISTERS: Alternately twist your hips side to side as you skip over the rope. This is more challenging than you think—the tendency is to move your arms as you twist side to side, which can really mess up your rhythm. Focus on twisting your hips *only* while your arms turn the rope normally. This one trains both your coordination and your brain, as it requires a lot of mental focus.

Schoolyard Routine

Time: 20 minutes

This is one of my favorite routines, and every time I do it I have fun and smile. I was inspired by the games I used to play as a girl. For me it brings back that feeling of freedom and worry-free life!

Your goal here is 20 solid minutes of exercise, and as you get more fit, you can work your way up to 25 or even 30 minutes. As with the Level I workouts, take breaks when you need them for recovery, stay hydrated, and let yourself have some fun.

What You'll Need

water

towel

The Plan

Put on an up-tempo cardio playlist and make sure you have plenty of room. This routine will last for about 5–7 songs, depending on their length. You should be exercising for about 20 minutes total.

THE MOVE	THE REPS	THE MUSICAL COUNT
Hopscotch	4 Right	4
Hopscotch	4 Left	4
Double Dutch	2 Right	4
Double Dutch	2 Left	4
Reach Around the World	2	8
Leapfrog	4	8
Kick and Move	4	8
Fast Feet	2	16

footwork options

You can do this routine two different ways. You can either use both feet equally (as it's described below), or you can do one side at a time, starting with your right foot for round 1 and switching to your left foot for round 2.

AND REMEMBER: You don't have to stick to the 8-count sets. That is only my suggestion for putting together a dance. Since this is *your* workout, you can do as many reps of each move as you like, just so long as you're moving continuously and breaking a sweat.

Hopscotch

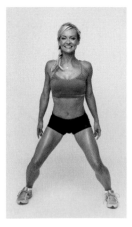 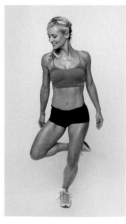

Stand on one foot with your opposite knee bent, heel lifted behind you, and your arms at your sides [1]. Hop on one foot [2], moving forward a few inches with each hop. Switch feet and repeat. Do 4 reps, each leg (4 counts).

LOW-IMPACT TIP: Instead of hopping, march in place, bringing your knees up high to waist level and swinging your arms. Do 4 reps, each leg (4 counts).

Double Dutch

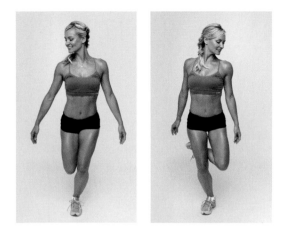

Stand with your feet wider than shoulder-width apart, arms at your sides [1]. Hop and bring your right heel up behind you by bending your knee and trying to kick your right glute [2]. Hop and put your foot back down. Switch legs and repeat. Do 2 reps, each side (4 counts).

LOW-IMPACT TIP: Stand with your legs wider than hip-width apart and squat down, making sure your knees are over your toes. Extend your legs and stand back up, simultaneously lifting one heel behind you, bending your knee, and trying to kick your glute. Switch legs and repeat. Do 2 reps, each side (4 counts).

Reach Around the World

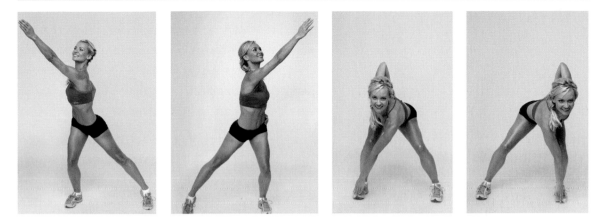

Stand with your feet wider than your hips, your knees slightly bent, and your arms bent and ready in front of you. Reach up high to the right diagonal with your left hand [1], pull your arm back in, then over to the left diagonal with your right [2] and pull it back in. Reach down to the right toe with your left hand [3] and pull it back in, and finally to the left toe with your right [4] and pull it back in to complete one repetition. Do 2 reps (8 counts).

Leapfrog

Stand with your feet wider than hip-width apart. Reach both arms up into the air and jump off the floor a few inches [1]. Land softly, bending your knees and immediately crouching down, reaching your hands toward the ground between your feet [2]. Explode back up to leap off the floor again, and repeat the sequence. Do 4 reps (8 counts).

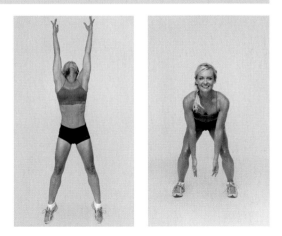

LOW-IMPACT TIP: Instead of jumping into the air, reach to the floor with both hands, then alternately lift one knee to hip height as you stand back up. Do 4 reps (8 counts).

Kick and Move

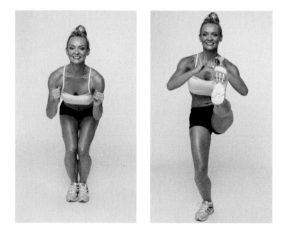

Stand with your feet together, fists at your shoulders, elbows bent and tucked into your sides [1]. Kick forward at hip height with your right foot [2], then hop your feet together and jump back a step in retreat. Do all reps on one side before switching to the other.

Fast Feet

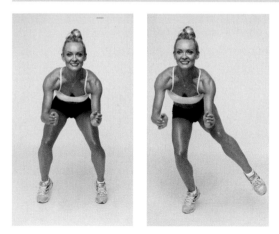

Stand with your feet wide, your knees bent, and your hands and arms held in front of you in a crouching "ready" position [1]. Get up onto the balls of your feet. Run quickly in place [2], keeping your weight centered as your feet move.

Level III: Principal

CARDIO WORKOUT

As a Principal dancer, you are a pivotal part of a performance: all eyes are on you, watching your every move. It's a lot of pressure, but you can handle it—and do you know why?

Because you're strong, capable, and ready for the challenge! Head into this Principal cardio routine with confidence and power.

Jump Rope III

Time: 15 minutes

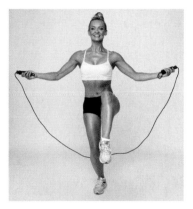

As a Principal exerciser you should be able to jump rope continuously for at least fifteen minutes. You're an animal! But of course, you can still take little breaks when you need to; just don't stop moving. Use the footwork options to challenge yourself. I like to do a minute of each option to change things up. It makes the time fly. . . .

footwork options

JUMP JACKS: Alternately jump your feet apart and then together while skipping the rope.

SPLIT JUMPS: Start with one foot forward and one foot back. Jump the rope and switch feet in midair so you land with your feet in the opposite positions.

HIGH KNEES: "Run" in place, alternately lifting your knees to hip height while skipping over the rope with each turn. You can even try actually running while skipping, hopping the rope with each step. This is pretty fun—if you have the space, you should try it!

Football Routine

Time: 30 minutes

Whether or not you're a football fan doesn't matter—you'll get a great workout with this high-energy routine. You're pretty much an expert exerciser now, so you should be good to go for at least 30 minutes of continuous cardio. If you have the time and inclination you can tack on a few more songs and make it a 45-minute session, or you can stick with 30 minutes and increase the intensity instead. Make the moves bigger or bolder, jump higher or squat lower. Anything that ratchets up the intensity will also increase the calorie burn!

What You'll Need

water

towel

The Plan

Get ready to rumble! Do this routine for the duration of about 10–12 songs, or roughly 30 minutes' worth of exercise. Once you get the routine down, add your own personal touches, and have fun.

THE MOVE	THE REPS	THE MUSICAL COUNT
Clear the Field	4	8
Heel Retreat	4	8
Clear the Field	4	8
Heel Retreat	4	8
Tornado Twist	8	8
Split Jump and Reach	4	8
Skip Jump	1	8

Clear the Field

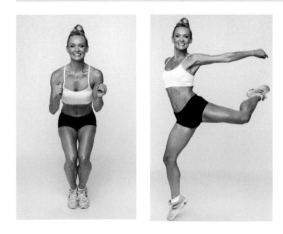

Stand with your feet and knees together, arms at your sides. Leap to your right, sweeping your arm across your body as if to move an opponent out of your way, and bring your left leg up behind you, knee bent [1]. Land softly on both feet and repeat to the opposite side to complete one repetition [2]. Do 4 reps (8 counts).

Heel Retreat

Stand with your feet together, fists under your chin, with your elbows bent and tucked into your sides [1]. Hop backward on your left foot, simultaneously extending your right foot in front of you, flexing it and tapping the heel on the floor [2]. Jump your feet back together and repeat, alternating sides. Do 4 reps (8 counts).

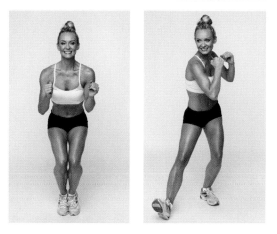

Tornado Twist

Clasp your hands together in front of your chest, arms extended parallel to the floor. Hop and twist your hips to the right while twisting and pulling your arms to the left [1]. Continue, alternating sides [2]. Do 8 reps (8 counts).

LOW-IMPACT TIP: Instead of jumping and twisting your hips, tap your heel out to the side while extending your arms to the opposite side. Do 8 reps (8 counts).

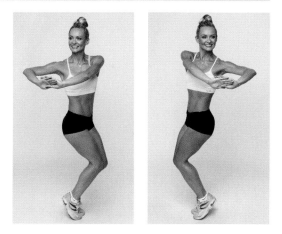

Split Jump and Reach

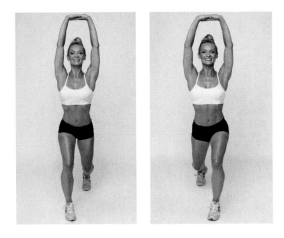

Stand with your feet together and clasp your hands in front of your thighs, arms straight [1]. Jump your feet apart, bringing your right foot forward and your left foot back. Simultaneously reach your arms overhead [2]. Jump your feet back together, bring your arms back down, and repeat, alternating sides. Do 4 reps (8 counts).

LOW-IMPACT TIP: Alternately lunge-extend your back leg behind you into a lunge while raising arms up and lowering back down. Do 4 reps (8 counts).

Skip Jump

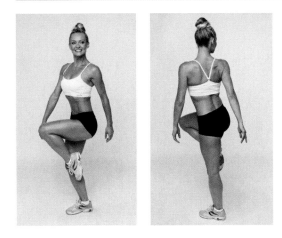

Skip forward four times, then backward four times [1, 2], changing direction smoothly with each switch. Do 1 rep (8 counts).

Chapter 9
Stretching Your Limits

Dance, when you're broken open. Dance, if you've torn the bandage off. Dance in the middle of the fighting. Dance in your blood. Dance when you're perfectly free.

—RUMI

I've never met a dancer who wasn't super flexible, but just like the rest of us, they didn't start that way! They work at it, and work at it hard, practicing their flexibility each and every day. When I was a professional dancer, I always made sure to cool down and stretch properly after every rehearsal and performance. In all my years, I never sustained a serious injury, and I strongly believe that my diligent flexibility routine was a big part of that enduring health.

Most people are very tight in certain areas of their bodies, especially the hips, neck, and back. This is usually due to a lot of sitting, either at a desk for work, driving in a car, or kicking back on the couch, relaxing. If you've had an injury in the past, you might also notice that you have tightness there or in the surrounding area, which is usually due to a buildup of scar tissue around the site of the injury. As we age, many of us will also experience arthritis, which causes pain and stiffness in hips, knees, and back.

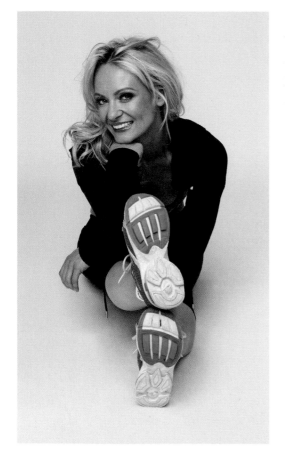

Fortunately, flexibility is something you can regain with patience, time, and consistent effort. Becoming more flexible has so many benefits—from alleviating pain to preventing injury to increasing your range of motion and enabling you to move with ease, both in exercise and everyday living.

Stretching is also an important part of recovery—it's like a little detox session to clear your mind and clean out your system. Gentle stretching allows your muscle fibers to release and flush out built-up lactic acid—a metabolic waste product of exercise that can get trapped in cells and cause stiffness and soreness. Breathing deeply as you stretch also helps you relax physically and mentally, and delivers oxygen to your tissues, which can improve circulation and accelerate the time it takes you to rebound from a workout. A post-workout stretch also helps you mentally transition back into your day. When I stretch, I like to focus on specific muscles, consciously asking them to relax and elongate and thanking them for a job well done. It's a really great way to connect with my body on a different level.

After every BBS workout you should spend at least 10–15 minutes stretching. For every stretch you want to go to the limit of your range of motion—which can be a little uncomfortable—but not push yourself to the point of pain. Hold the stretch at that sweet spot of resistance for 30–60 seconds, slowly relaxing and increasing your stretch while inhaling and exhaling deeply. There's no bouncing here—only slow, deep stretches that lengthen and release your muscles, better allowing them to recover and be ready for your next workout.

Everyone has a different level of flexibility and the tightness of our muscles is impacted by the other activities we do. For example, if you jog or run regularly, you might have tight hips and hamstrings, so spend a little extra time working on them. Or if you enjoy cycling, your quadriceps might need some TLC. Whichever areas feel the stiffest or sorest are the ones you should give the most love. The more time you devote to your flexibility routine, the more results you will see. It's a good idea to note your improvements in your journal as you go along so you can track your progress. Maybe you were barely able to touch your toes initially, but after 6 weeks you can place your palms on the floor in front of you. That's a major accomplishment—write it down!

The Stretches: All Levels

TIME: 10–15 MINUTES

A dancer's body is her computer, her office, her only tool for work, and she must take care of it both onstage and off. Do this stretching routine after every BBS workout to properly nurture your body, helping it recover, progress, and grow.

Standing Side Stretch

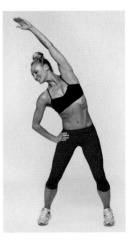

Stretches: obliques, shoulders

Stand with your feet hip-width apart. Place your left arm on your left hip and reach your right arm overhead, stretching it diagonally toward the left side of the room as you bend at the waist. Hold for a few moments, or until you feel the stretch in you obliques. Repeat on your left side.

TIP: Make sure to keep your hips square: try to avoid twisting them to one side or the other.

Q&A

QUESTION: Can I stretch before I work out instead of after?

ANSWER: Yes, but with this caveat: do the stretches described in this chapter at the end of your session. These are called "static" stretches and are designed to lengthen and relax your muscles, increase your range of motion, and improve flexibility. You don't want your muscles to be too relaxed when you're getting ready to exercise, so if you want to stretch beforehand, do more "dynamic" stretches, movements that simultaneously warm you up and improve your range of motion, such as twisting side to side, swinging your arms or legs, and moving your limbs around in all directions to loosen up and get them ready to work. You never want to stretch a cold muscle, so dynamic stretching is perfect for pre-workout flexibility.

QUESTION: Back when I used to dance we were told to bounce when we stretched to make our muscles stretch farther. Is that still okay?

ANSWER: That sort of "ballistic" stretching is no longer recommended. Ballistic stretches force your muscles to stretch beyond their natural capacity, which can cause tearing and straining, especially if a muscle is cold. Static stretching, as described in this chapter, has replaced ballistic stretching for post-workout flexibility training. Through slow, gentle release and deep breathing, your muscles stretch safely and effectively to improve your range of motion and accelerate recovery time.

QUESTION: My right hamstring is a lot tighter than my left, but I have never had an injury. What gives, and how can I make both legs even?

ANSWER: It's pretty normal to be tighter on one side than another. Whether you favor one side while you sit without realizing it, or are simply built a little off kilter (most people are not perfectly symmetrical!), this is totally normal. No one's body is perfect, but you can work to bring both sides into balance. Spend a little extra time on the parts that are tightest and need more attention.

Standing Calf Stretch

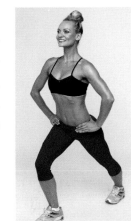

Stretches: calves, ankles

Stand with your feet apart in a wide lunge, with your back leg straight and your front knee bent. Press your rear heel toward the floor and hold. You can place your hands on your hips or hold on to a wall for balance if need be. Hold 30–60 seconds.

TIP: Slowly bend and straighten your rear knee, rolling up onto your toe, then pressing your heel back down again to stretch your foot, ankle, and calf.

Standing Quad Stretch

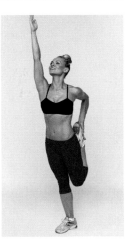

Stretches: Quadriceps

Stand with your feet hip-width apart. Bend your right knee and bring your heel toward your glute. Grab the toe of your shoe with your right hand and hold. You can place your left hand on a wall or a sturdy chair for balance if need be. Hold 30–60 seconds; repeat with left leg.

TIP: Make sure your bent knee is pointing straight down toward the floor; don't let it flare out to the side. Also make sure you're not overarching your back. Keep your pelvis tucked underneath you to keep your spine safe.

Chest and Shoulder Stretch

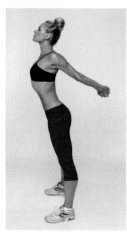

Stretches: pectorals, front deltoids, rotator cuffs, biceps

Stand with your feet hip-width apart and reach both arms behind you. Lace your fingers together and straighten your arms. Keep your chest lifted and press your shoulders down away from your ears. Hold 30–60 seconds.

TIP: If you can't lace your fingers together, hold a rolled-up magazine behind you with your hands as close together as you can get them. As you stretch, try to slowly "walk" your hands in toward each other to deepen the stretch.

Cat/Cow

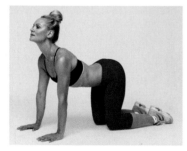

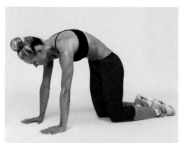

Stretches: abdominals, hip flexors, back, neck

Start on your hands and knees—in tabletop position. Lift your chin and look up, dropping your belly toward the floor, arching your back, and lifting your tailbone to the sky to make the cow position [1]. Hold here for several breaths, then drop your head, round your back and tuck your tailbone under to make the cat [2]. Continue, alternating slowly between the two for 60 seconds.

TIP: Imagine your spine as a whip of licorice—bendy and soft and flexible!

Downward Dog

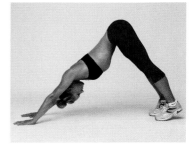

Stretches: calves, hamstrings, glutes, shoulders, upper back, chest, neck

Start in plank position with your hands directly underneath your shoulders and your head, hips, and heels in line. Lift your hips up toward the ceiling and shift your weight back, dropping your heels toward the floor and your head between your hands. Your arms and legs should be straight and your body should make an inverted V. Hold for 60 seconds.

TIP: Breathe deeply, and sink into your heels with each breath, and lift your tailbone on each exhale. You can also spread your fingers wide on the ground for better balance.

Cobra

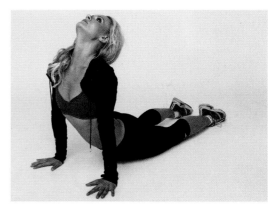

Stretches: lower back, abdominals

Lie facedown on the floor with your legs straight. Place your hands on the floor at shoulder level and, pressing down into the floor with your palms, slowly push your upper body up from the floor, pressing your hipbones toward the floor and lifting the abdominal muscles toward your spine.

TIP: Don't let your shoulders creep up to your ears. Push them down and away as you stretch, relaxing the shoulder blades to avoiding creating tension in the back and shoulders.

Seated Hamstring Stretch

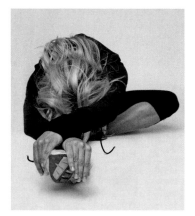

Stretches: hamstrings

Sit on the floor with your legs extended in front of you. Fold your left leg in toward your pelvis, keeping your right leg straight and both hips on the floor. Reach your hands forward toward your right foot and slowly fold your body over your right leg, reaching as far toward your toes as you can while keeping your left hip on the floor. Switch legs and repeat.

TIP: Don't worry about being able to touch your toes right away, just reach as far as you can! Also remember to try to maintain a flat back, even though it's tempting to hunch over.

Stretching Playlist

I love to use music to relax and wind down from my workout. Here's a playlist I suggest to do just that.

"Sparks," by Coldplay

"Wonderwall," by Ryan Adams

"Teardrop," by Massive Attack

"Falling Slowly," by Glen Hansard & Marketa Irglova

"Hallelujah," by Jeff Buckley

"Let It Be Me," by Ray LaMontagne

"More Than Words," by Extreme

"Ordinary People," by John Legend

"Gavin's Song," by Marc Broussard

"Burn for You," by John Farnham

The Plan

Suggested Stretching Routine

STRETCH	TIME
Standing Side Stretch	30–60 seconds, each side
Standing Calf Stretch	30–60 seconds, each leg
Standing Quad Stretch	30–60 seconds, each leg
Chest and Shoulder Stretch	30–60 seconds
Cat/Cow	60 seconds
Downward Dog	60 seconds
Cobra	30–60 seconds
Seated Hamstring Stretch	30–60 seconds, each leg

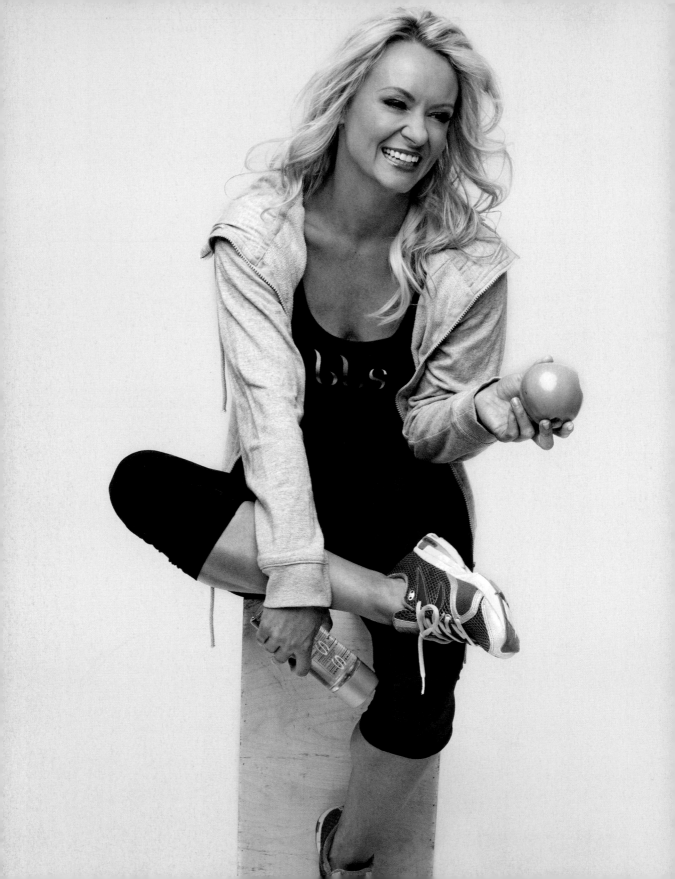

Fuel Your Fire

Chapter 10
Eat to Win

To dance is to be out of yourself. Larger, more beautiful, more powerful.

—AGNES DE MILLE

Disordered Eating

Growing up, I witnessed firsthand how eating disorders such as anorexia and bulimia made many of my peers mentally and physically ill, draining them so much that they didn't have the strength left to dance. Fortunately, my mum made sure that I always ate well and stayed healthy, so I never fell into that trap. She taught me how to make healthy eating a lifestyle, and I encourage my clients and students to do the same.

I don't believe in dieting or starving yourself to lose weight: not only are those practices usually unhealthy, but they are also only effective in the short term. Unless you're going to be on a diet for the rest of your life, you're just going to go back to your former way of eating and likely gain back any weight you've lost. Eating whole, nutritious foods has to become a daily habit. For many women this is a difficult shift to make—we've been sold so many crazy weight-loss ideas that it seems too simple when I tell them that it's not as much about how much, when, where, or why they eat as simply *what* they eat. It's really so simple, but it's the very thing that trips most of us up. The other variables all fall into place when you consistently choose to eat whole, nourishing foods. That's it.

The key is to learn to eat healthfully each and every day, focusing on clean and, whenever possible, organic foods. This is the fuel that will give you the nutrients, energy, and strength you need to accomplish your daily activities and your workouts, and to feel good in your body and mind. After a while, eating healthfully will become something that you value and embrace because it offers so many benefits—from weight loss to increased energy to better digestion to a clearer mind.

I've put together a basic plan to help you get started on the path to nutritious eating. As I've said, I don't believe in diets, but I do believe that we all need a little help when we're starting something new—so consider this plan to be just that. It is straightforward and easy to follow, and the recipes are simple and delicious. (Trust me, I'm not one to spend much time in the kitchen, but I am a girl who likes yummy food.) So let's get started.

The Plan

Most weight-loss plans involve calorie counting, which is something I simply don't believe in. I know that some people like the structure of calorie-based diets, as it allows them to "budget" their food, but I don't believe we should look at food as something to budget. To me, "budgeting" calories means your view of food is already skewed in an unhealthy way, because the implication then is that food should be rationed very carefully, and that you can "spend" your calories on things that are good for you or "save" them for splurges. Calories aren't like money! Saving up to buy a fabulous pair of shoes is healthy behavior. Saving up a day's worth of calories to "spend" on pizza and ice cream is not. When you look at food in terms of calories, you don't learn how to eat properly and nourish your body. To be healthy and to really lose weight and keep it off, you've got to adopt a new way of thinking about food.

My plan will help you do this in a few ways:

* We'll cover how to choose the foods that are best for your health and your weight-loss goals, and look at why they're so great.

- I'll give you tips on how to grocery shop, what foods to buy, and how and what to eat when you're out.
- We'll look at how to prepare healthy, nutritious meals for yourself and your family. I'll also offer some guidance on meal planning and portion control.

If you follow these simple guidelines, I can promise that your body and your brain will feel energized, your skin will glow, and, yes, you'll lose weight. Let's start with getting to know the very basic units in our food that can either help us or hurt us: the nutrients.

Nutrient Know-How

It's probably been a while since you learned about macronutrients and how they work in your body, but this knowledge is essential to knowing how to eat healthfully. So let's have a quick review, shall we?

Protein

It's important to get enough protein when you're working out, as protein is used to build muscles. Your body also needs protein to create enzymes, form hormones, and perform many other bodily functions. We get protein from both the plant and animal foods we eat on a daily basis. Beef, pork, poultry (turkey, chicken), seafood, and dairy (yogurt, cheese) are good examples of animal-based sources of protein, while soy products, beans, seeds, nuts, and some grains are good examples of plant-based proteins.

Because your body cannot store protein or amino acids like it does carbohydrates and fat, you have to provide your body with a continual supply. Each meal or snack you eat should contain a protein so you get plenty of amino acids with which to build that fat-burning muscle and repair your tissues after your workouts. Protein also adds satiety to a meal, meaning it makes you feel full for a longer period of time. This translates to less between-meal snacking and energy slumps.

All animal proteins and some plant proteins are considered "complete," meaning they contain the full spectrum of the nine essential amino acids available in nature.

It's important to get all nine of these amino acids each day to build and repair your muscles and tissues and keep your body running smoothly. Most plant-based proteins are considered "incomplete," meaning they are missing one or more amino acids. Combining two incomplete proteins, such as beans and rice, can create a complete protein, so vegetarians and vegans can still get enough amino acids by being mindful of these important combinations.

In my experience, women often don't get enough protein in their diets. I am not sure exactly why that is, but it seems to be a typical issue with many of my clients. But I promise if you add protein to each meal and snack you have, it'll make that meal "stick to your ribs" and you'll be better able to adhere to your plan.

My favorite proteins:

free-range chicken

wild-caught fish

grass-fed beef

tofu

black beans

egg whites

chickpeas

Greek yogurt

Carbohydrates

Even though they have been vilified by diet books, weight-loss plans, and women's magazines, believe it or not, carbs are a necessary part of your diet. Carbohydrates provide the energy you need to fuel your workouts and daily activities as well as to promote healthy brain function. There are two basic kinds of carbohydrates: simple and complex. Simple carbs are usually processed foods that have been stripped of their natural fiber and many of their other nutrients. These include things like bread, rice cakes, table sugar, cereal, pasta, and crackers. Your body is able to quickly break down these kinds of carbs into glucose—or, sugar—and if you eat a lot of them, they can trigger drastic blood-sugar fluctuations as your body tries to handle a sudden spike in glucose. This can give you a heady rush of energy, followed shortly thereafter by a hard crash when that glucose disappears.

Complex carbs, on the other hand, are whole foods that still contain their natural vitamins, minerals, and fiber. These include items like oatmeal, brown and wild rice, and other whole grains, as well as fruit and vegetables. Complex carbs take longer to break down, so the glucose is released into your blood in a slow, steady stream, which prevents the crash and burn effect of simple carbs. Complex carbs also contain fiber, which provides bulk and roughage to maintain your digestive system and keep you regular. I am a big proponent of eating as many whole foods as possible, and my nutrition plan is based on this premise.

I recommend planning what kinds of carbs you eat—and when—according to your energy needs throughout the day. For example, if you exercise in the morning, you might have some whole-grain cereal with almond milk or a piece of fruit to supply you with solid energy about an hour before your workout. If you're typically relaxing in the evening, skip the simple and starchy carbs and go for the vegetables, since your energy requirements are lower and you won't be as likely to store those extra carbs as fat. And, yes, you can eat potatoes, bread, and white rice; just time them properly. The ideal time to have simple carbs is post-workout, when you are depleted of blood sugar. Your body is looking to replenish those stores, and will use the carbs from the simple sugars you ingest to do that rather than storing them as fat.

My favorite complex starchy carbs:

sweet potatoes

brown rice

yams

apples

oatmeal

whole-wheat bread

citrus fruits

My favorite complex fibrous carbs:

kale

spinach

broccoli

cauliflower

mushrooms

squash

green beans

asparagus

quinoa

My favorite post-workout simple carbs:

rice

mashed potatoes

crackers

juice

pasta

Did you know that your brain runs exclusively on glucose? If you're having trouble focusing in the middle of the day, have a snack containing a complex carbohydrate, like an apple or a piece of whole wheat toast with almond butter to get your brain back on track.

Fats

Hey, don't knock fats—healthy fats are an important part of any weight-loss plan. Yes, you read that right: you should *eat fat to lose weight*. Fats come from both plant and animal sources and include foods like oils, nuts, cheese, and avocado. Fats break down into fatty acids in the body, which provide energy, transport fat-soluble vitamins (vitamins that can only be carried to cells and organs when they attach to a fatty acid in the bloodstream), and keep your skin and hair glowing and healthy. Like protein, fats also provide satiety to a meal, so when you add a little bit of a healthy fat, like olive oil or avocado, to a meal, you will feel fuller and more satisfied.

You know I don't believe in counting calories, but it is important to note that fat is more energy-dense than the other macronutrients. In fact, fat contains about twice as many calories per gram as protein or carbs. So the key thing with fats is to eat the right ones, and in the right portions.

While healthy fats are an important part of your diet, there are other fats that have no place in your meals: saturated fats and trans fats. Saturated fats are found naturally in animal products like cheese, meat, whole-milk dairy, and egg yolks, as well as in plant sources such as palm and coconut oils. Having an excess of saturated fat in your diet can clog arteries and blood vessels, cause weight gain, and raise your cholesterol. To keep your intake of saturated fats to a minimum, buy lean cuts of meat, trim the skin from poultry, and avoid whole-fat dairy products.

Trans fats begin life as regular fats, but are then chemically altered in a process called "hydrogenation." During this process, a liquid vegetable oil is heated and combined with hydrogen. The result: a very stable product that, when added to processed foods, helps them last a long time on a shelf without spoiling. Trans fats are found most often in foods that contain partially hydrogenated oils such as processed baked goods, doughnuts, taco shells, and chips. Trans fats may increase the lifespan of processed foods, but they do *not* do the same thing for our bodies. In fact, they're a double-trouble whammy for your cholesterol, raising the bad LDL molecules and decreasing the good HDL ones. This leads to an increased risk of heart disease, which is the number-one killer of both men and women! The good news is that the FDA is starting to catch on to the health effects of these foods. Shortly before this book went to press, the FDA announced that partially hydrogenated oils are no longer recognized as "safe." This may be an important first step in banning these nasty substances altogether!

My favorite healthy fats:

avocado

olive oil

all-natural peanut butter

raw nuts (almonds, walnuts, cashews)

raw seeds (sunflower, chia, sesame)

flaxseeds

sesame oil

Buzzword

Another name for trans fats is "partially hydrogenated oil." When you read the ingredients listing on a food label and see these words, put the item back on the shelf and walk away!

Q&A

QUESTION: Organic foods are so expensive. Is it really that important to buy organic?

ANSWER: I often get this question from my clients, since I urge them to choose organic food whenever possible. First, let's look at the definition of "organic." Organic foods have been grown and/or raised without the use of chemicals and pesticides. As a result, they are a bit more labor-intensive to produce, and they are often grown or raised in smaller quantities—which means that they cost more (per unit) to produce.

The designation of organic matters more in some cases than others. For example, in the case of fruits that have a thick peel that you don't eat—such as oranges or bananas—conventional is fine. But for meats and poultry, as well as for produce such as lettuce, spinach, grapes, apples, or strawberries, where you eat the whole plant or fruit with the skin, I recommend buying organic. If you're unable to buy organic fruits and vegetables, try to be extra diligent about washing your produce. Try some of the "cleaning" products they sell in the grocery store, such as the scrubbing brushes or veggie "soaps." These do a decent job of cleaning off the residual chemicals and pesticides that stick to nonorganic produce, but of course nothing can replace a food that is grown cleanly and naturally.

For more information on the use of pesticides and a list of which fruits and veggies to buy organic, check out the Environmental Protection Agency's information page: www.epa.gov/international/toxics/pop.html.

Caveman Cuisine

You may have heard about the Paleo (short for Paleolithic) diet in the media lately, as it is gaining widespread popularity. I know I said I don't believe in diets or gimmicks—and I don't—but the fundamentals of my eating plan are similar to this style of eating.

Why? Because the Paleo lifestyle advocates eating only those foods that were available when our cave(wo)man ancestors roamed the planet—those that we either hunted or gathered. Our ancestors didn't have Wonder Bread or Pop Tarts or Hot Pockets. They foraged for fruits and vegetables and nuts and seeds, and hunted animals to provide themselves with sustenance.

Research shows that our hunter-gatherer ancestors didn't suffer (at least not in great numbers) from the kinds of illnesses that plague modern society, such as obesity, Type 2 diabetes, and heart disease. While I'm not suggesting you need to go into the wild and spear your own water buffalo to stay disease free, I do think there is a powerful lesson to be learned from the Paleo philosophy: if we eat closer to the land, as early man did, we can satisfy our nutritional needs while managing our weight effortlessly and lowering our risk profile for disease.

My eating plan is much less restrictive than what is advocated in many Paleo diet books. I don't believe, for example, that you need to cut all grains from your diet (early man had not yet learned to grow, harvest, and process wheat—so most wheat products are forbidden in strict Paleo diets). Here are the guidelines upon which I base my eating plan:

- HEALTHY PROTEINS: Protein should comprise about 30% of your overall diet. I advocate a balance of plant and animal protein, as animal protein often contains saturated fat. I recommend eating some protein with each meal and snack.

- PLANT-BASED, HIGH-FIBER CARBOHYDRATES: Slow-digesting, fiber-rich carbs like fruits and vegetables should make up about 45% of your diet. I'm not saying that you can never eat another slice of bread or another cracker again, but definitely opt for whole-grain versions of these with as few ingredients as possible. Remember, eat higher-starch foods to power your activities—you want to eat those foods to fuel workouts, but not at night, when you're sedentary. They provide your body with a lot of energy, and if you don't burn it off, it is stored as fat.

- MODERATE FATS: Healthy fats should comprise 25% of your diet. Remember to choose monounsaturated fats. The majority of your fat intake should come from plants—like nuts, seeds, oils, and avocados; and from fatty fish, like salmon and mackerel. You want to limit your intake of animal fats in the form of red meat, poultry skin, and full-fat dairy products.

- LOW SODIUM: Our predecessors may have used salt to preserve perishable foods, but they certainly didn't put it in a shaker and douse every meal with it. High sodium intake is associated with a slew of diseases and illnesses, including hypertension, heart disease, and strokes. With my plan you'll reduce your sodium intake and increase your water intake—which will flush out any excess sodium lingering around.

- NUTRIENT-DENSE FOODS: Cavemen needed energy to hunt, gather, build, run, and survive in the wild. It was essential for them to eat nutrient-dense foods that would fuel their cells, provide sustained energy, and boost their immune systems. When you eat more whole, unprocessed foods, you are eating the stuff of life—vitamins, minerals, and antioxidants—all of the things that give our bodies health.

Q&A

QUESTION: The Paleo diet sounds good in theory, but I don't eat a lot of animal protein. Will this work for me?

ANSWER: You don't need to be a ravenous carnivore to follow this eating plan. Seafood is a great source of protein if you're not a huge meat eater. Wild-caught salmon and tuna, shellfish, sardines, and mackerel are all very nutritious sources of protein. A little free-range chicken here and there goes a long way as well—plus, it's easy to prepare and keeps well in the fridge. If you are 100% vegetarian, you can easily meet your daily protein requirement with plant-based proteins such as vegetarian protein powders, beans, nuts, tofu, quinoa, Greek yogurt, and legumes. Just be aware of the fat and carbohydrate content in vegetarian dishes—you don't want to overdo it!

Chapter 11
The Guidelines

When you dance, you can enjoy the luxury of being you.

—PAULO COELHO

Now that we've been over the basics of nutrition and the philosophy of my eating plan, let's put information into action. My plan is built on ten basic guidelines that are meant to be incorporated into your overall lifestyle and inform your attitude about food. This isn't a plan that tells you exactly what to eat every single day, but rather one that educates you and empowers you to make the food choices that are best for your body and lifestyle. Remember—food is not your enemy. It contains the nutrients and energy you need to live and dance and think and thrive!

Guideline 1: Learn Proper Portions

Each meal or snack you have during the day should contain a combination of protein, carbs, and fat. While I am not an advocate for strict portion control by measuring and weighing every ounce of food you prepare, I do recommend learning how to eyeball portions so that you can avoid overeating. Here are a few basic rules of thumb:

- PROTEIN: A serving size of protein should be about the size and thickness of the palm of your hand. This is a good measure because everyone's hands are different, and so you eat in accordance with your body's size and its needs. I, for instance, do not need the same portion of protein as a professional football player!

- FAT: Aim for a serving size roughly equal to the size of a golf ball for solid fats like avocados or nuts, or a tablespoon for liquids such as olive oil.
- STARCHY CARBS: One serving of starchy carbs is about the size of your fist. Think of a half cup of cooked rice, a slice of whole-wheat bread, or a medium-sized piece of fruit.
- FIBROUS CARBS: A healthy serving size of fibrous carbs is roughly the size of two open hands. Imagine half a head of lettuce resting in there.

When preparing a meal at home, try to use these guidelines as a reference. A snack is about half the size of a meal, so simply divide each meal portion in half for the perfect quantity.

Get the idea? It's not too complicated, and there's no need to make it so. Be intuitive and smart with your choices and I guarantee you'll eat healthfully. You know deep down what is good for you and what is not. Follow your instincts—you know when your gut is right, and when it is tempting you down the wrong path.

Guideline 2: Eat Mini-Meals

For those of you who are used to eating two or three times a day, it might take a little bit of time to adjust to this guideline. But know this: to lose weight you need to eat more. Personally, I eat all day long. Not huge meals, mind you, but rather 4–6 small meals and snacks throughout the day. I graze like a cow! This system keeps me energized and fueled for my active schedule all day long, and I am never hungry.

Breaking your daily food intake into 4–6 small meals and snacks will do several good things for you. First, it will provide your body with a continual stream of fuel, so you'll never be starving or experience an energy slump. This means you'll be more likely to stick to your plan and less likely to binge on junk foods and sugar when you're overly hungry or tired. Eating more frequently will also boost your metabolism. Think of it like this: your metabolism is a fire, and when you put more wood on it, it burns hotter. If you deprive it of wood, it dies out. Continually supplying your metabolism with fuel means it is always burning hot, incinerating fat and burning calories.

To make the most of your meals, spread them out evenly through the day. For example, if you get up around 7 a.m. and have breakfast, your next meal or snack should be around 10 a.m., then lunch around 1 p.m., another snack around 4 p.m., with a final meal around 7 p.m. Make sense? Basically you're adding wood to your fire every 3–4 hours, keeping your blood sugar steady and even, and your metabolism roaring!

Guideline 3: Think Ahead

It might sound like a lot of work to prepare and eat so many little meals, but it's actually pretty easy; all it takes is a little planning. I recommend taking one day during the week to cook and prep a bunch of food. Make big batches of protein, like roasted chicken, ground turkey, and hard-boiled eggs ahead of time. Put some of it in the fridge and some of it in the freezer for later in the week. It's also handy to steam a batch of brown rice, lentils, or quinoa, or bake some yams or sweet potatoes to eat for a week. These store and reheat nicely. Another thing I recommend is buying a bunch of fresh veggies and fruits at the farmers' market and cutting them up right away. Put them in easy-to-see glass containers in the fridge where they are visible, so you can easily use them for meals and snacks.

If you know that you're going to have an especially busy week and won't have the time to prep lots of fresh produce, buy some prechopped veggies, bagged lettuce, or ready-to-eat fruit. All of these are available at the grocery store in the produce section. Also check out the lovely grilled protein options at stores like Whole Foods, and buy a few precooked options that you can grab quickly and throw in a salad or pair with some whole grains. The better prepared you are, the less likely you'll be to hit the drive-thru.

Once you get all your food prepped and ready to go, plan your meals and snacks for the week. It always helps me if I actually write it out, so I don't overeat one day and shortchange myself the next. And you'll be surprised how easy it is to make a meal when the ingredients are already cooked, chopped, or prepped! The easier it is, the more likely you are to stick to your game plan. Invest in a small, portable cooler and pack your food to take with you to work, to your kids' soccer games, or wherever life takes you day to day.

Q&A

QUESTION: What if I am so busy one day that I miss a meal or snack?

ANSWER: It's not the end of the world, but when you do finally get to have a meal, eat slowly and drink lots of water. When I am starving, I eat my veggies and protein first to make sure I get those in before I hit the starchy carbs! But do your best to try not to let that starvation happen in the first place. Carry small, portable snacks with you—such as raw nuts or fruit—in case you get stuck in a work meeting, in traffic, or at the doctor's office. Life happens, but if you're prepared, it makes sticking to your plan a whole lot easier.

Guideline 4: Eat Breakfast— No Excuses. (Seriously.)

Okay, now I am going to be your mum for a second: Breakfast is the most important meal of the day—so you'd better start eating it if you're not already. Period. No excuses!

Since you probably ate dinner around 6 or 7 p.m., and likely get up around 6 or 7 a.m., that's twelve full hours you've gone without eating. If you then skip breakfast and wait it out until lunch, that's another five or six hours without food, and by now you're literally *starving* yourself! How likely are you to make healthy food choices when you're starving? Not very likely. So, please—*please*—eat your breakfast. Even if it's something small—a piece of fruit and a hard-boiled egg, or a smoothie—breakfast will reignite your dying metabolic fire and give you energy right away.

Q&A

QUESTION: I get up at the crack of dawn, and I just can't stomach food that early in the morning. What should I do?

ANSWER: I have so many clients with the same problem! Sometimes it's hard to have a whole meal early in the morning, but it's so important to start your day with energy. Even if you don't have an appetite in the morning, I still recommend having something small: a few slices of an apple with a little peanut butter; a handful of raw nuts; or a half a yogurt with some sliced banana. It might take you a few weeks to get used to eating that early, but eventually you will adjust. And remember that a few hours later you should be eating again, this time a more substantial meal that contains all your food groups for optimal nutrition!

Guideline 5: Don't Skip

Many women believe that skipping meals leads to faster weight loss, but in fact it works the opposite way: if you're not providing your body with a constant intake of good, healthy fuel, your metabolism actually slows down, causing you to store more fat.

Starving yourself can also lead to binge eating. By the time you do allow yourself to eat, it's hard to resist plowing through that whole bag of potato chips. In the end, you'll feel defeated, both physically and emotionally. Trust me: skipping meals is never a good way to lose weight. Stick to the all-day grazing to ignite your metabolic fire and lose weight the healthy way.

On the flip side, if you miss a meal or a snack, don't make the mistake of doubling up on your calories at your next meal to make up for the one you missed. Your body can only handle so many calories at once, so an overdose of food at one meal means that any excess that is not used to feed cells and power metabolic functions will be stored as fat.

Guideline 6: Focus on the Whole

In the next chapter I'll share a sample grocery list that will help you get started on this plan. But, really, you don't even need a list of specific foods, you just need to know one thing: Eat Whole Foods.

As we've discussed, whole foods are foods that are as close to the source as possible—the kinds of foods our cave sisters ate. Whole foods are generally not packaged; they don't come in a box or wrapped in layers of plastic. They have been minimally processed, which means that they haven't been refined or chemically altered. Whole foods aren't injected with sugar and salt and artificial flavorings. They still contain their natural fiber, vitamins, and minerals, and thus offer your body nourishment and energy.

One of the great things about eating whole foods is that because they contain all of their nature-given fiber, they are more satisfying and filling than processed food (which has been stripped of its natural fiber), so you are less likely to overeat. I mean, think about it—it's pretty easy to eat a bag of chips or a box of crackers, but how easy would it be to eat a bag of apples? You probably couldn't get through more than two because you would have a stomachache.

Whole foods never contain ingredients you can't pronounce. Read the ingredients label for any product before you buy it. If you see something you don't recognize and can't pronounce, don't eat it!

Guideline 7: Drink Water

Your body is made up of roughly 70% water, and even a 1% dehydration level can wreak havoc on your system. Every cell in your body needs water to function properly, and water is involved in nearly all the biochemical reactions that take place within a cell. If you are dehydrated, you could actually be impairing your cells' ability to metabolize glucose, which means you'll potentially be burning fewer calories! Because your body cannot manufacture water itself, you must drink it or get it from the foods you eat. Water is responsible for a variety of functions in the body, including:

- liver and endocrine function
- flushing toxins and wastes out of the body
- regulating body temperature
- aiding digestion
- cushioning your organs and joints

Drinking plenty of water is not only essential to your overall health, it's also important when you're trying to lose weight. First of all, water helps you metabolize food, making it easier to break down and digest, enabling you to better extract the nutrients. Water also helps you feel full, so when you're eating a meal or snack, take a few bites, then have a few sips of water.

Proper hydration also means less bloating. Water helps flush out excess sodium from your tissues that causes the bloat, so while it seems like it should be the opposite, drinking *more* water actually means you retain *less* water!

Most of your hydration should come from drinking plenty of plain old H_2O. I recommend at least a half gallon a day, more if you can manage it. On days when you exercise, you should drink even more to counteract the water you lose through breathing, sweating, and an increased metabolic rate. Have about 1–2 glasses 30 minutes before you work out, sip water frequently during the workout, and follow up with another 1–2 glasses afterward. Be sure to keep track of your water intake by noting it in your journal. At the end of the day, tally it all up to see if you made it to the half-gallon mark.

Good sources of water (besides your tap!):

raw vegetables

raw fruits

leafy greens

herbal tea

decaf green tea

almond, soy, or rice milk

green juice

coconut water

Did you know that your body sometimes interprets dehydration as hunger? When you find yourself craving a salty snack or a sweet treat, first drink a large glass of water. Wait 20 minutes and see if your cravings subside.

Q&A

QUESTION: I drink a lot of iced tea during the day. Does that count toward my water intake?

ANSWER: Yes and no. Coffee, tea, and some sodas and energy drinks contain caffeine, which is a diuretic. So while you're certainly getting some liquid with these beverages, you're also expelling more than you would normally because of the caffeine. I always recommend having a glass of water for every caffeinated beverage you drink to counteract its diuretic effect. If you can, find an iced tea you like that contains no caffeine, or even make your own. And be sure that the tea is unsweetened tea—some iced-tea mixes contain as much sugar as a handful of chocolate! I like to brew ginger tea, which makes a lovely iced tea, and in the summer iced mint tea is a cool and refreshing drink.

Bored with Plain Water? Try These Ideas!

- Add fresh strawberries or cucumbers to a pitcher and chill in the fridge.
- Pour in a packet of Emergen-C.
- Squeeze in a fresh lemon or lime.
- Try sparkling water instead of still.
- Add a splash of unsweetened cranberry or pomegranate juice.
- Use half water and half coconut water.

Guideline 8: Mind Your Sodium

Sodium is a tricky little beast. It is found naturally in a lot of foods, but these days, an abundance of salt is added to just about everything—cookies, cakes, breads, restaurant meals. You name it, it's got extra salt.

Your body does need sodium to function properly: it helps the nervous system transmit impulses, tells your muscles to contract, and helps regulate your fluid levels. But too much sodium has been linked to high blood pressure, stroke, and other heart problems. It can also leach calcium from your tissues and bones, which can contribute to osteoporosis.

The Food and Drug Administration recommends that women consume no more than 2,300 milligrams of sodium daily. Let's put that into perspective: two teaspoons of soy sauce contains around 670 mg of sodium; a serving of pretzels can contain as much as 1,715 mg of sodium; and just seven olives contain around 1,556 mg of sodium—that's nearly 10% of your daily allowance per olive! Sodium adds up quickly.

Because you get plenty of sodium in the foods you eat naturally, there's no need to use your shaker. If you're at a loss for how to season your food to add flavor, check out page 202 for a list of suggestions. Also, read the labels on any packaged or processed foods you buy to check the sodium content, and when you go out to eat, ask that your food be prepared without added salt. I guarantee if you cut back on your sodium you'll feel lighter, less bloated, and more energized.

Foods naturally high in sodium:

saltwater crab (1,072 mg per 100 g)

fresh (not frozen) shrimp (244 mg per 100 g)

celery (96 mg per 120 g)

chard (77 mg per 36 g)

eggs (71 mg per large egg)

beets (64 mg per raw beet)

ocean-caught tuna (43 mg per 85 g)

carrots (42 mg per one medium)

spinach (24 mg per 30 g)

Five Easy Ways to Cut Sodium from Your Diet

- Eat fresh vegetables instead of canned.
- Cook your own chicken and turkey for sandwiches instead of using lunch meat.
- Use low-sodium chicken, vegetable, or beef stock when cooking.
- Make your own salad dressings and marinades instead of buying bottled.
- Avoid Chinese takeout; when you do order, ask for the sauce on the side and use only sparingly. Never order from a restaurant that uses MSG (monosodium glutamate, a form of sodium to which many people are sensitive or even allergic).

Guideline 9: Have Your Cheats and Treats

Anyone who knows me knows I can't live without my chocolate! Everyone deserves a treat now and again, and denying yourself constantly can lead to feelings of deprivation and to binge eating down the line.

I recommend eating as healthfully as you can six days a week, and having one cheat meal on day seven to take the edge off. This is how life in the real world operates, after all. No one eats perfectly all the time! Take yourself out to a nice restaurant, order a delivery pizza for a cozy night in, or have a glass of wine and share a dessert with girlfriends—whatever you're craving. Make the most of your meal, dessert, or cocktail. Eat or drink it slowly, savor every bite, and have no guilt.

My top five favorite treats (can you tell I love sweets?):

a glass of French Champagne

ham-and-cheese croissant

a Nutella crepe

chocolate peanut butter ice cream

Lindt milk chocolate with hazelnuts

Guideline 10: Imbibe Wisely

I love a nice glass of wine now and then, but truth be told, alcohol contains a lot of empty calories and can slow your metabolism and digestion significantly. When you drink alcohol, your body sees it as a toxin and puts all other digestion on hold until it handles the alcohol. I recommend looking at alcohol as a treat or a cheat, and having it only once or twice a week at most. Here are a few tips for choosing your adult beverage and incorporating it into your plan:

- Choose light beer over regular.
- Use sparkling water and a squeeze of lemon or lime as a mixer instead of soda, juice, or tonic.
- Avoid anything colorful and blended that comes with an umbrella—unless you're in Hawaii on vacation! A 4.5-ounce piña colada, for example, can contain around 30 grams of sugar, and a 20-ounce mudslide (like the ones you see at every chain restaurant) can contain as much as *80* grams.
- Pick red wine over white to benefit from its antioxidant properties.
- Skip liqueurs, ports, and dessert wines, which contain tons of sugar.
- Sip your cocktail slowly and enjoy it!

Plan of Action

You may be saying to yourself, *These guidelines seem too simple, there has to be a catch!* But there's no catch; and, yes, they are simple. But if you follow them and make them part of your daily routine, you will give your nutrition a complete overhaul, be healthier, and lose weight—I promise!

You don't have to implement all of these guidelines at once, overnight. Take them one at a time, if you like, and ease into this healthier way of eating. Once you've successfully mastered one, move on to the next one. If you're a fast-acting kind of person, try one or two a day; if you need more time to adjust, implement one new change every week. There's no absolute here, but remember that the quicker you make changes, the quicker you will get results!

Chapter 12
My Cleanse

We must always change, renew, rejuvenate ourselves; otherwise we harden.

—GOETHE

What Gives?

Okay, I know what you're thinking: *Simone just gave us guidelines for
healthy eating and now she's telling us to go on a cleanse? What gives?!?*

It's true that many commercially available cleanses involve starvation or meal-
skipping, but that's not how mine works at all. My cleanse is inspired by a good friend
of mine, Dr. Frank Lipman, a renowned, highly in-demand holistic medical practi-
tioner based here in New York City. I read his book *Spent* in one sitting and simply
went mad about his approach, which he calls "restorative eating."

Let me preface this: I was a typical New Yorker, running around all the time, busy
as a bee. I ate on the go in between classes and clients and never had regular meal-
times. I was always starving because I would wait too long to eat, then would stuff
my face with whatever was convenient. I had fallen off the healthy food wagon and
was making bad choices again and again. I felt tired, irritable, and sluggish, and no
amount of coffee or napping could make me feel better. So when I read in *Spent* that
eating the right foods could restore my health and vitality, I was sold.

The premise of restorative eating is this: you eliminate the foods that are irritating and exhausting to your system and replace them with whole, nutritive foods. In doing so, you detox your organs, boost your ability to heal, and improve your general sense of well-being and health and—most appealing to me at the time—gain loads of energy.

Replacing foods that irritate your digestive system with whole foods can also help reduce inflammation in the body. Inflammation is an immune reaction—your body's attempt to remove harmful elements from your system and heal itself. Many people have food sensitivities or allergies—typically to things like gluten, sugar, or dairy—which cause this inflammatory response, and replacing these foods with whole, nutritive things can shut off this response and return your body to a healthy, energetic state.

So, book in hand, I turned myself into a human guinea pig and tried Dr. Lipman's cleanse on for size. It was incredible! I ate a ton of food, had loads of energy, and my skin was radiant. My hair and nails grew long and healthy, and I even lost a few pounds as a bonus.

Here are some of the many incredible benefits of cleansing:

Rests the digestive system.

Balances and maintains healthy gut bacteria (called your "microbiome").

Decreases inflammation.

Cleans out the digestive tract and eliminates toxins from the body.

Supports healthy liver function.

Every now and again when I'm feeling a bit sluggish or run down, I do the cleanse over again—but I've made a few modifications along the way to better suit my needs. So when I was writing this book, I knew I wanted to let you in on this "celebrity secret" by sharing my version of the cleanse with you.

NOTE: Though it is not necessary to do this cleanse in order to succeed with the BBS program, I do recommend you consider it seriously. It only requires a commitment of two weeks, and you stand to gain a lot of knowledge about yourself, your body, and your nutritional sensitivities if you give it a go.

Q&A

QUESTION: What is a cleanse?

ANSWER: Simply put, a cleanse is a system of eating in which you allow your digestive system to "rest" for a specific amount of time. This is accomplished through dietary means, by eliminating toxic and allergenic foods and replacing them with healthful, whole foods and drinks.

QUESTION: What is detoxification?

ANSWER: Like cars, our internal engines are subject to waste buildup and can become sluggish over time. These waste products, or toxins, can come about from stress, an overproduction of hormones, or from the foods we eat. Detoxification through cleansing can help bring your body back into balance by decreasing the amount of toxins you take in, while boosting your body's ability to eliminate those toxins already in existence.

What Toxins Can Do

- Interfere with the normal production and action of hormones. Hormones regulate things such as weight, reproductive health, metabolism, and your immune system, but the presence of toxins can prevent them from properly functioning, causing you to gain weight, become ill, or even become infertile.

- Attach to and alter chromosomes, which can cause birth defects, as well as cancer in people of all ages.

- Overstimulate or block enzyme activity. Enzymes are tiny biological molecules responsible for thousands of chemical reactions that happen within your body on a daily basis. For example: digestion. Enzymes are released into the stomach to help break down food into smaller particles so their nutrients can be more easily absorbed. Toxins can affect digestion by causing an overproduction of acid in your stomach and giving you heartburn, or by inhibiting digestive enzymes from doing their job so your food is not properly broken down and assimilated.

Cut It Out

So how does one do this fabulous cleanse? It's actually quite simple: for two weeks you will eat specific, healthful foods that will nutritionally support your body's natural detoxification system. You'll feel lighter, more energetic, and more mentally focused when you're done, and chances are you'll also lose a little weight to kick-start your BBS journey.

I am also going to ask you to give up a few things you might find challenging to abandon. But it's important that you cut out these foods completely, and here's why: many people are sensitive or even allergic to foods and don't even know it. Cutting out specific foods on a temporary basis will help you get in tune with your body and will allow you to really pay attention to how your body reacts to those foods.

For example—maybe you're a dairy addict. You don't really think about how much dairy you're eating on a regular basis, but after a scoop of ice cream, a piece of cheese, or a bowl of cereal with milk, you always feel bloated. When you're eating these foods you barely think about your swollen belly—you just assume it's normal, that it's how you're built. But when you do a cleanse and you eliminate an ingredient like milk, you can monitor how your body reacts and really notice the difference when you exclude it from your diet. That's one of the many benefits of cleansing: learning which foods trigger unhealthy responses in your body.

Many foods are highly allergenic. Sometimes your sensitivity is mild, causing feelings of fatigue, but other times it could be strong, giving you digestive issues or even joint pain. So here are the biggies you're going to cut out: caffeine, sugar, dairy, and gluten. Let's talk about each of these and why it's a good idea to leave them out of your diet, even if it's only temporary.

Caffeine

Caffeine is an artificial stimulant, and it's highly addictive. It's so addictive, in fact, that many people experience withdrawal symptoms (headaches, fatigue) when they stop drinking it. But I encourage you to give it up for two weeks and see how you feel. If you are a several-cups-a-day kind of person, I recommend weaning yourself off gently rather than going cold turkey. Try following the plan below for a week before starting your cleanse:

- Day 1: Have one regular cup of coffee. If you have a second one, blend 50% regular with 50% decaf.
- Days 2–4: Have one or two cups of 50% regular, 50% decaf.
- Days 5–6: Have one cup of 25% regular and 75% decaf.
- Day 7: Substitute weak green or black tea for coffee.

Why you should avoid caffeine:

There are many reasons to cut out caffeine. One is that it dehydrates your muscles and tissues, making you less able to perform your best while you're working out. Your body may interpret that dehydration as hunger, causing you to snack or overeat when all you really need is some water. Caffeine can also interfere with sleep patterns, especially when consumed close to bedtime. A well-rested body is a healthy, fat-burning body. In fact, some recent research uncovered that when you're sleep-deprived you're more likely to store calories as body fat! Furthermore, you're more likely to make poor food decisions when you're tired, reaching for that quick burst of energy in the form of a processed carb or sugary treat. Cutting back on your caffeine habit helps to ensure that you fall asleep and stay asleep easily at bedtime.

Caffeine also increases heart rate and blood pressure, can promote feelings of nervousness, and, when consumed in excess, can cause indigestion and headaches. So what are you waiting for? Overhaul your morning routine and begin to wean yourself off of your daily buzz. After a week or two you'll feel more energetic than you ever did after a double latte.

Red Alert

Dark chocolate does offer many health benefits, but it also contains a lot of caffeine. The higher the percentage of cocoa solids (which is typically advertised prominently on the label), the more caffeine it packs. Though the content varies between manufacturers, an average bar can contain about 40 mg of caffeine, which is about the same as a cup of tea. By comparison, the same sized milk-chocolate bar contains only about 10 mg. This doesn't mean that you should cut out dark chocolate altogether (or that you should eat milk chocolate—which is full of sugar and dairy products), but it does mean you should abstain from dark chocolate while on the cleanse and avoid eating it late at night in general.

Buzz-o-Meter

BEVERAGE/FOOD	CAFFEINE CONTENT*
coffee, regular brew (8 oz.)	95–200 mg
semisweet chocolate chips (1 cup)	104 mg
espresso (1 oz.)	40–100 mg
Red Bull (8.4 oz.)	76–80 mg
Mountain Dew (12 oz.)	46–55 mg
Diet Coke (12 oz.)	38–47 mg
tea, green (8 oz.)	30–60 mg
tea, black (8 oz.)	20–90 mg
Coca-Cola (12 oz.)	30–35 mg

*Numbers are approximate. When coffee and tea are brewed longer or stronger, their caffeine content will increase.

Sugar

I admit that I am somewhat addicted to sugar—I could eat it for breakfast, lunch, and dinner, and I am not alone. Americans consume tons of sugar every year: the average American consumes 152 pounds of sugar a year. That's three pounds of sugar a week, or 42.5 teaspoons a day.

But how can that be? you might be asking. *I don't eat sweets or drink soda!* Here's the thing: added sugars are hiding in a lot of foods where you might not expect them, like in salad dressings, crackers, bread, cereal, yogurt, and even harmless-looking condiments like ketchup. As a matter of fact, sugar is the number-one ingredient added to foods in the US.

Decreasing or eliminating the amount of processed food in your diet will definitely help cut down the amount of added sugar you consume, and becoming a conscientious label-reader is a must when you do purchase packaged foods. The American Heart Association recommends that women get no more than 100 calories a day from added sugar from any source. So when you read a food label, look for total grams of sugar and keep a running tally in your food journal.

Sugar Aliases

Sugar comes in a variety of names on food packaging. Here's a list of sugar aliases to look out for:

agave syrup	fructose	high-fructose	molasses
brown sugar	fruit juice	corn syrup	sorbitol
corn sweetener	concentrate	honey	sucrose
corn syrup	glucose	lactose	syrup
dextrose		maltose	

Added sugars aren't the only form of sugar lurking in the food you eat—fruit and fruit products are often loaded with sugar as well, though the sugar in fruit is a naturally occurring sugar called fructose. While I would always opt for natural sugars over added sugars, the truth is that any form of sugar can cause weight gain. When given the choice, eat a piece of whole fruit rather than having fruit juice, canned fruit, or fruit jams, compotes, and spreads. The whole fruit contains fructose but it also contains fiber, which slows down the digestion process and helps counteract the insulin response your body will generate in response to the fructose.

Why you should avoid sugar:

Refined sugar, that white stuff in your sugar bowl, has no nutritive value, meaning it offers your body only empty calories. But here's the thing: sugar is your body's preferred source of fuel. When you digest carbs, you break them down into simple sugars called glucose, which your body then uses to fuel your brain and muscles. This is great, and the system works well—until you eat *more* sugar. Excess sugar is stored quickly in your tissues, first as glycogen—energy to be used later—but then, when you don't use all of that energy, it gets stored as fat.

Eating an abundance of sugar will also give you that oh-so-lovely sugar high . . . followed, shortly thereafter, by an equally horrific crash. This up-and-down blood-sugar roller coaster damages your hormonal balance as well as your pancreas, which produces and regulates insulin. Eating an abundance of sugar over an extended period of time can lead to a variety of diseases, such as metabolic disorders and even Type 2 diabetes.

It's typical to crave sugar if you haven't eaten enough food at a meal to provide the fuel your body needs, or if you've waited too long to eat between meals. Your body is hungry and it's looking for a fast way to get some nutrients, so it tells you, *Eat that candy bar! It will really help me with my energy level, and hey, it tastes great!* Eating small meals and snacks all day long will allow you to keep your cravings under control, and keep your energy level balanced.

Still not convinced? All of the following health effects are linked to consuming too much sugar:

- increased risk of diabetes, obesity, and heart disease
- excess accumulation of fat in the liver, causing inflammation and damaging the liver tissues
- elevated levels of anxiety and hyperactivity
- suppressed immune system and increased inflammation in the body
- increased incidence of tooth decay
- increased triglycerides in the body from excess sugar and alcohol calories, both of which are linked to heart disease and obesity

Surprising Sources of Added Sugar

bacon	canned fruit	flavored soy and	peanut butter
barbecue sauce	crackers	almond milk	salad dressing
bottled spa-	energy bars	instant oatmeal	sports drinks
ghetti sauce	fat-free foods	ketchup	teriyaki sauce
bread	flavored alcohol	lunch meat	

Q&A

QUESTION: What is high-fructose corn syrup and why is it so bad for you?

ANSWER: HFCS (for short) is a corn syrup that has been chemically altered so that it tastes sweeter. Food companies use it because it's a cheap source of added sugar. It is used in many packaged foods, though prime examples include soft drinks, cereal, and condiments. As HCFS has become more abundant in our food sources, the level of obesity has skyrocketed, leading some to the conclusion that HFCS is more harmful than regular sugar and affects weight gain by altering our normal appetite response. The jury is still out on this issue, but I would avoid it whenever possible. Anything that is so chemically altered can't be good in my book.

QUESTION: What about artificial sweeteners? Can I have any of those to satisfy my sweet tooth?

ANSWER: There are tons of fake sugars around, and they are all composed of chemicals. I'm not a huge fan of these sweeteners since they are so unnatural, and would advise skipping them altogether. There are plenty of available, all-natural alternatives to sugar, such as stevia, honey, and agave nectar, all of which can be used in cooking and baking.

How Much Sugar Are You Eating?

DRINK/FOOD	SUGAR CONTENT
Skittles (14 oz. 1 bag)	47 g
Coca-Cola (12 oz. 1 can)	39 g
orange juice (fresh, 8 oz.)	20 g
Hershey Bar	19 g
Gatorade (8 oz.)	14 g
whole orange (medium)	13 g
Frosted Mini-Wheats (1 cup, dry)	11 g
Cheerios (1 cup, dry)	1 g

Dairy

Dairy is a staple in most everyone's diet, and it's long been viewed as healthy and essential to the development of strong teeth and bones. How many of us grew up in a household where we had to finish our glass of milk before we could be excused from the dinner table? As kids, we were taught that milk was good for us. But these days we're learning more and more that dairy products are not an essential part of a healthy diet.

Cows are ruminants, and should be feasting on green grasses as their main dietary staple. Unfortunately, today most dairy cows are fed a diet of soy, corn, and other commercial feeds that contain lots of things, but no fresh grass. This changes the nature of their milk, and therefore how humans digest it.

In addition, these cows are often given large doses of hormones and antibiotics to make them grow bigger and prevent illness, which also affects the quality of their milk. Our milk is then pasteurized, which is necessary since milk produced on massive commercial dairy farms could contain harmful bacteria, but that processing also destroys valuable enzymes and vitamins. After the pasteurization process the milk is homogenized, another refinement that creates an end product that is even harder for humans to digest. This homogenization can also trigger an immune response in the body, causing inflammation.

Urp! Signs of Dairy Sensitivity

Millions of people are lactose intolerant, meaning they cannot digest and break down lactose, the main protein found in milk, and millions more are dairy-sensitive. Not sure if you have a dairy intolerance or sensitivity? Check out the list of common symptoms below and see if any of them are a match for you:

respiratory problems

excessive mucus production (having
   a chronically stuffy nose, needing
   to clear your throat a lot, etc.)

gas, bloating, or diarrhea

fatigue

joint pain

rashes

acne

And, finally, all of that nutritional information drilled into our heads as kids didn't really give us the full picture when it comes to the health benefits of milk. Yes, milk contains calcium, but so do green vegetables, nuts and seeds, and tofu. I highly recommend cutting out dairy for life, but if you can't face giving up cheese—which I totally understand!—at least give it a try for the cleanse. You might be surprised at how you feel after eliminating dairy from your diet for two weeks. And if it does turn out that you have a sensitivity, the good news is that there are so many alternatives available these days—from soy ice cream to goat's milk yogurt to rice, almond, soy, and coconut milk—you will have plenty of options to get your needed dairy fix.

Non-Dairy Calcium Sources

FOOD	CALCIUM
tofu	406 mg per ¼ block, or 116 g
kale	101 mg per one cup
edamame	98 mg per one cup
sesame seeds	88 mg per tbsp
almonds	75 mg per oz
broccoli	43 mg per one cup, chopped
molasses	41 mg per tbsp
figs	18 mg per one medium fig

Q&A

QUESTION: Are eggs considered a dairy product?

ANSWER: No. While they might be shelved in the "dairy" aisle at the grocery store, they are not made from cow's milk and are not a dairy item.

QUESTION: How are almonds and rice made into "milk"?

ANSWER: It's actually pretty simple—simpler than milking a cow, in fact! You can even do it at home. For almond milk, soak almonds in water for 24 hours, then drain and blend the nuts with fresh water until completely pulverized. Strain this pulp with a fine strainer and you've got almond milk. For rice milk, take one part cooked rice and four parts water, blend together, then strain for rice milk. So easy and so healthy!

Gluten

Gluten has certainly become a hot topic these days. It seems like every time you turn on the TV or read a magazine, someone is talking about its ill effects. But what is gluten anyhow, and why is it "dangerous"?

Gluten is a protein found in grains and seeds such as wheat, barley, rye, and spelt. Wheat is the worst offender, as gluten comprises more than 90% of its proteins. Since wheat is found in nearly everything, including breads, pastas, condiments, and baked goods, it's estimated that the average American ingests more than 150 pounds of gluten a year!

While only about 1% of the population has celiac disease—a severe allergy to gluten in which the body's reaction to even a small amount of gluten can be life-threatening—it's estimated that nearly 30% of people have an intolerance to gluten on some level and don't even know it. These people don't produce the enzyme needed to break down gluten, and this undigested protein can leak through the gut wall and get into the bloodstream. When this happens, the immune system kicks into gear, responding to the leaked protein as if it were a dangerous foreign agent. The inflammatory and autoimmune responses that arise from gluten sensitivity can impact almost any organ system, including your brain, muscles, skin, bones, liver, heart, and endocrine system. These responses tax your body and can lead to chronic feelings of unwellness.

Doing this cleanse can help you determine if you're among the 30% of the population who suffer from some level of gluten intolerance or sensitivity. Cutting out gluten for two weeks will give your digestive and immune systems time to rest and recover. If you feel better afterward, chances are you're somewhat intolerant. After the cleanse, reintroduce gluten into your diet slowly and see how you feel. If your symptoms return, you're probably intolerant.

Not sure how you're going to live without bread? Try these gluten-free alternatives to wheat:

Symptoms of Gluten Intolerance

early menopause

fatigue and lethargy

impairment in mental functioning and/or depression

infertility

nausea, gas, bloating, diarrhea, constipation, and/or abdominal pain

numbness in the extremities

rashes, itching, blistering

recurrent canker sores

weight loss or gain

amaranth	potatoes	sorghum
buckwheat	quinoa	tapioca
corn	rice (wild, brown,	
millet	basmati)	

Surprising Sources of Gluten

Gluten is found in some unlikely places. Check out some of these hidden sources!

beer	Communion	marinades	soy sauce
chicken-stock	wafers	matzo	spice blends (i.e.,
cubes	envelope glue	Play-Doh	taco mix)
cold cuts	gin	shampoo	stamps
	lipstick	soup	

Gluten Aliases

Gluten has many names in the food-processing industry. Read your labels carefully to see if your product contains any of the terms below. If it does, then it contains gluten:

couscous	hydrolyzed veg-	modified food	semolina
flour	etable protein	starch	texturized vege-
graham	kamut	natural flavoring	table protein
	malt	seitan	

Q&A

QUESTION: What is celiac disease?

ANSWER: Celiac disease is a genetic allergy to gluten. Gluten triggers an immune response in the small intestine that can wear away the lining of the intestine and prevent it from properly absorbing nutrients. Over time this can cause malnutrition, anemia, weight loss, stunted growth, loss of bone density, and other potentially life-threatening symptoms. The most common symptoms are diarrhea and weight loss, but many people experience no symptoms at all until they become quite sick. The only way to know if you have this disease is to get tested by a doctor.

The Cleanse Eating Plan

Now that we've gone over the four major offenders that you will eliminate for two weeks—caffeine, sugar, dairy, and gluten—let's focus on what you'll be replacing these nasties with: fresh, delicious, wholesome foods that will nourish and energize your body and your mind. You do not have to worry about going hungry on this cleanse!

While the cleanse officially lasts for just two weeks, it will be helpful if you take an extra week beforehand to start weaning yourself off of these foods slowly. If you go cold turkey, you'll feel awful, especially if you consume a lot of foods containing these substances daily. Here are a few tips for the week *before* your cleanse.

Cleanse Cheat Sheet

- Start cutting back on caffeine. Use the box on page 158 as a guideline.
- Begin replacing processed foods with whole foods.
- Eat more fresh produce, such as veggies and fruits.
- Eat more protein, especially fish and chicken.
- Cut your gluten intake in half and eat more whole grains.

- Reduce the amount of added sugars you consume.
- Prep yourself mentally for the next two weeks, thinking positive thoughts about how great you'll feel instead of dreading the deprivation.

Week 1

Now, I am not going to lie, the first few days of this cleanse might prove a little challenging. You may feel more tired, more bloated, and perhaps even a little nauseous, but this is only temporary. Your body is ridding itself of toxins. Once these poisons are out of your body you will start to feel better day by day. By the end of two weeks you'll be flying! Here are some tips for making the first week a bit easier:

- Drink lots of water to help flush out toxins and wastes.
- Nap if you can find the time.
- Exercise to get your blood moving and help your body eliminate toxins.
- Write in your journal what you're eating, what you're not eating, and how you feel each day.
- Don't give up—it will get easier!

Week 2

If you've stuck to your guns, you're probably feeling pretty darn good right about now. You're most likely sleeping better, feeling more energized, and thinking more clearly. Your digestion has probably also improved—you feel less bloated and gassy, and if in the past you suffered from heartburn or indigestion, those have also likely been alleviated. Here are a few things to remember as you come into the homestretch:

- Keep drinking lots of water. Hydration is essential not only in Week 1, when you're eliminating toxins, but all the time!
- Continue exercising.
- Continue to note in your journal about what you're eating, not eating, and how you're feeling.
- Try a few different foods from the grocery list on page 182. Now is a good time to see how your body reacts to them in a clean, open state.

Post-Cleanse

The week after your cleanse is also a crucial time: here you'll be reintroducing the foods that you cut out for the last several weeks—if you want to, that is. You may have found that you're sensitive to something and don't want to eat it anymore. But if you do decide you can't live without your bread, milk, sweets, or coffee, here are some tips for reintroducing these foods properly:

- Add foods back into your diet slowly, *one item at a time*. Eat that food at breakfast, then check in with yourself the rest of the day to see how you feel.
- Note your reaction to that food. Do you still feel energized, or do you feel sluggish after eating it? Do you have a headache or an upset stomach after eating it?
- If your reaction is neutral or positive, then you probably are not sensitive to it. If it is slightly or dramatically, then you probably have a sensitivity or an allergy to it.
- If you suspect you have a strong allergy, make an appointment to see your doctor.

Life After Cleanse

The idea behind this cleanse is to help you reset your body and give you insight into which foods help you look and feel your best. If you eliminated and then reintroduced one of the foods I suggested with no reaction whatsoever, you are probably not sensitive to it and can eat it with no issues. The goal here isn't to create paranoia or guilt about what you eat—but to educate and empower you to make the best possible choices moving forward.

The Plan

Okay, enough talking—time to cleanse! Because I don't like to "prescribe" a diet for anyone, I am instead going to outline a cleanse I myself have done, including what I ate for breakfast, lunch, dinner, snacks, and a few desserts for each of the 14 days I was on it. This is simply an example of how all the information you've just been given can come together into a nutritious, energizing meal plan. Use my cleanse as a template to help you formulate your own, swapping in foods you prefer over my choices using the grocery list on page 182, but sticking to the same basic premise: clean, whole foods eaten throughout the day. Good luck!

DAY 1

Breakfast

Oatmeal with almond milk, topped with raisins, dates, and prunes

Lunch

Small bowl of vegetable soup

One slice of rye bread with almond butter

Snack

Carrots and celery sticks with a small serving of hummus

Dinner

Quinoa Tabouli Salad with chickpeas and almonds (recipe, page 193)

DAY 2

Breakfast

Medium bowl of chopped fresh fruit (orange, pineapple, and mango) topped
with a small handful of toasted pumpkin seeds

1 cup decaf herbal tea

Lunch

4 pieces each of tuna and salmon sashimi

One large scoop of hummus with cauliflower, cucumber sticks, celery, and
radishes

Snack

1 handful of raw almonds

Dinner

Roasted Herbed Tilapia Filets (recipe, page 195)

Mixed green salad with walnut dressing

DAY 3

Breakfast

Grilled tomatoes on 1 slice gluten-free bread, toasted

Lunch

Sliced avocado and a small handful of walnuts over mixed greens with balsamic vinaigrette

1 orange and a handful of grapes

Snack

2 rice cakes with 2 teaspoons of honey

Dinner

Wild rice with toasted pumpkin seeds

1 grilled organic chicken breast

Big side of grilled mixed vegetables

Dessert

Handful of raspberries and half an apple, sliced

DAY 4

Breakfast

Banana Berry Smoothie (recipe, page 189)

Lunch

1 baked potato

Large mixed salad with toasted almonds and balsamic vinaigrette

Sliced pear and orange sections

Snack

Kale chips with figs and almonds

Dinner

Quinoa sprinkled with chopped toasted cashews

Spicy Spinach and Mushrooms (recipe, pages 198–199)

DAY 5

Breakfast

Raw Muesli with rolled oats, almonds, flaxseeds, apple slices, and fresh berries
(recipe, page 191)

Lunch

Veggie-and-Rice Frittata (recipe, page 191)

Spinach, raspberry, and almond salad with olive oil and vinegar

Snack

1 banana

Dinner

Grilled organic chicken breast

Large kale salad with walnut oil dressing

DAY 6

Breakfast

Chocoholic Protein Smoothie (recipe, page 190)

Lunch

Quinoa Tabouli Salad (recipe, page 193)

Side of cubed watermelon with mint

Snack

2 handfuls of mixed nuts (pistachios, almonds, Brazil nuts, and hazelnuts)

Dinner

Salmon fillet with grilled peppers

Mixed green salad

Steamed green beans

DAY 7

Breakfast

Cinnamon Oatmeal with almond milk, and topped with chopped dates and figs (recipe, page 192)

Lunch

Small bowl of vegetable soup

2 rye crispbreads spread with guacamole and topped with chopped olives

Snack

Small bowl of fresh fruit (kiwi, grapefruit, and mango)

Dinner

Vegetable Curry over brown rice (recipe, page 196)

Dessert

Banana-Strawberry Sorbet (recipe, page 202)

DAY 8

Breakfast

Fresh-squeezed green juice (kale, spinach, and cucumber)

One slice toasted gluten-free bread spread with 1 teaspoon honey

Lunch

Spicy Chicken (recipe, page 197)

Side of fresh fruit (papaya and orange)

Snack

1 whole apple

Dinner

Rice pasta topped with lentils and tomato sauce

DAY 9

Breakfast

Fresh fruit muesli topped with grated apple

Fresh apple-and-orange juice

Lunch

Grass-Fed Beef Tacos (recipe, page 194)

Snack

1 rice cake spread with almond butter

Dinner

Chickpeas, cilantro, and lime over mixed greens

Dessert

2 Walnut-Date Balls (recipe, page 201)

DAY 10

Breakfast

Millet porridge with almond milk

Lunch

Turkey-Lettuce Sliders (recipe, page 194)

Side of fresh fruit (mango and pineapple)

Snack

1 handful of dried dates and apricots

Dinner

Small bowl of Simple Broccoli Soup (recipe, page 195)

1 organic chicken breast

Roasted Mediterranean Vegetables (recipe, page 196)

DAY 11

Breakfast

Pumpkin Pie Smoothie (recipe, page 190)

Lunch

Spinach Salad with Shrimp and Mushrooms (recipe, page 192)

Small handful of toasted almonds and pumpkin seeds

Snack

Raw broccoli, cauliflower, cucumber, and cherry tomatoes with hummus

Dinner

Roasted Herbed Tilapia Filets (recipe, page 195)

Side of Roasted Vegetables (recipe, page 198)

DAY 12

Breakfast

Oatmeal with rice milk, topped with chopped dates

Lunch

Rice pasta with tomato sauce and chopped vegetables

Smoothie with almond milk, mango, and banana

Snack

1 avocado halved and mashed on 2 crispbreads

Dinner

Vegetable Curry over brown rice (recipe, page 196)

DAY 13

Breakfast

Green juice with spinach, apple, kale, and cucumber

Lunch

Wild-Caught Sesame Salmon (recipe, page 197)

Parsnip and Sweet Potato "Fries" (recipe, page 199)

Snack

Smoothie with chocolate protein powder, banana, 1 tsp almond butter, and
almond milk

Dinner

1 medium bowl dairy-free pumpkin or sweet potato soup

Dessert

Cubed cantaloupe with mint

DAY 14

Breakfast

Banana Berry Smoothie (recipe, page 189)

Lunch

Turkey breast over kale and spinach salad with sliced avocado

Snack

2 tablespoons of hummus with carrot and celery sticks

Dinner

Falafel with large green salad, topped with pine nuts with balsamic dressing

Dessert

Chocolate Fudge (recipe, page 201)

Chapter 13
Food for Thought

Don't eat anything your great-grandmother wouldn't recognize as food.

—MICHAEL POLLAN

For most people, grocery shopping is a chore, but I actually love it.
Think of going to the grocery store as an adventure, and an opportunity to help
fuel your workouts, your goal to slim down and make your body as healthy and
strong as it can be. These days, grocery stores are well-stocked with a wide variety
of healthy ingredients, fresh organic produce, and high-quality proteins. Of course
they're also filled with thousands of packaged goods, a whole freezer case of temptation, and fresh-baked treats. Here are a few tips to help ensure grocery-store
success:

- MAKE A LIST AND STICK TO IT. Don't get distracted by special bargains or
  foods that used to tempt you. Remember your goals and purchase only what
  you came for.
- NEVER SHOP WHEN YOU'RE HUNGRY. This is a hard-and-fast rule of mine.
  When you're hungry, nothing looks better than chips, cookies, or candy.
  Have a meal or snack before you head to the store to stay focused on your
  intent.
- SHOP THE PERIMETER OF THE STORE. This is where most of the fresh, healthy
  things you will need reside.

- READ THE INGREDIENTS. If you're buying packaged goods, use this rule of thumb: if there are more than 5 things listed, and some of them you cannot pronounce or spell, don't buy it.
- EAT THE RAINBOW. Fruits and vegetables with deep, rich colors are high in vitamins, minerals, and antioxidants. Choose lovely produce in a variety of colors to get a full array of nutrients.
- WHENEVER POSSIBLE, BUY ORGANIC VEGETABLES, FRUITS, AND MEATS. As we discussed on page 138, it is a little more expensive, but it's worth it.
- BUY LEAN CUTS OF MEAT, SKINLESS CHICKEN BREASTS, AND FRESH FISH. These are all great sources of protein. Buy ocean-caught or wild-caught fish whenever possible.
- WHEN BUYING CANNED OR FROZEN GOODS, SHOOT FOR AS CLOSE TO NATURAL AS POSSIBLE. Choose low-sodium and no-sugar-added options; and remember, you need to be able to pronounce all of the ingredients on the label.

Deciphering the Labels

There's lots of label trickery going on these days. Food marketers recognize that consumers have become more savvy about their health, and you'll see lots of healthy-seeming promises emblazoned on their packaging. But not everything is as great as it claims to be. Here are a few tips to help you decipher real benefits from sneaky marketing tactics:

NATURAL OR ALL-NATURAL: This label is *supposed* to indicate that a food contains minimally processed ingredients and no artificial colors or flavors, but there is no legal definition for this terminology, and it is used liberally. For example, foods with GMOs can be labeled "all-natural." One could also argue that high-fructose corn syrup is all-natural, as it comes from corn. Be wary of this label.

ORGANIC: Organic foods must meet government-mandated regulations for being raised without the use of pesticides, hormones, or antibiotics. Products labeled as organic have an official seal and contain 95% or more organic ingredients.

MADE WITH ORGANIC INGREDIENTS: 70% of the ingredients must be organic; the other 30% are not regulated. These products cannot carry an organic seal.

SUGAR-FREE: The product does not contain sugar, but just because it is sugar-free does not mean it is calorie-free, and chances are it has a lot of refined flour and fats to make it taste good. It also likely contains artificial sweeteners.

NO SUGAR ADDED: These products don't contain *added* sugars, but they still can contain sugar. For example, a jam made only from fruit is naturally high in fructose. So even though no processed sugar has been added, it is still high in sugar.

NO GMOS: This product does not contain any genetically modified organisms or derivatives thereof.

FREE-RANGE: Meat or eggs with this label are produced from animals that were raised with access to the outdoors, rather than being penned up.

MADE WITH WHOLE GRAINS: A product can contain 99% processed grain and 1% whole grain and still make this claim! Hardly true, is it?

GRASS-FED: These cows are raised eating grass in a pasture instead of grains in a feedlot. A product (such as steak or milk) with this designation will be labeled "grass-fed" or "pasture-raised."

Q&A

QUESTION: What is a GMO?

ANSWER: A genetically modified organism, or GMO, is a plant or animal that has been engineered with DNA from bacteria, viruses, plants, or other animals to make it stronger, more hardy, or even resistant to pesticides. There is a big movement to ban the use of GMOs in the United States, or at least to require clear labeling of the products that carry them, and it is gaining momentum; but no legislation has passed yet for either cause. But in more than sixty countries around the world, including my homeland of Australia, there are restrictions or even bans on the production and sale of GMOs. Hopefully we'll get up to speed soon here, too!

Grocery List

I put together the following list to give you choices while you're on your cleanse and on my eating plan. Don't feel like you have to buy everything on this list! Choose what you already know you like, and use this as a guide for trying out new foods.

Herbs and Spices

anise	dill	red pepper flakes
arrowroot	fennel	rosemary
basil	garam masala	saffron
bay leaves	garlic powder	sage
black pepper	ginger	sea salt
caraway seeds	marjoram	tarragon
cardamom	mint	thyme
cayenne pepper	mirin	turmeric
celery seed	mustard powder	vanilla extract
cinnamon	nutmeg	whole grain mus-
coriander	oregano	tard
cumin	parsley	
curry powder	red chili powder	

Dry Goods

almond butter	extra-virgin olive	steel-cut or rolled
apple cider vin-	oil	oats
egar	flaxseed oil	unsweetened
balsamic vinegar	lentils	cocoa powder
beans (all types)	red wine vinegar	vegetable stock
capers	sesame oil	walnut oil
coconut oil		white wine vinegar

Grains

amaranth	millet	wild rice
brown rice	quinoa	
buckwheat	teff	

Condiments

- agave syrup
- balsamic vinegar
- low-sodium soy sauce
- mirin
- mustard
- red wine vinegar
- sesame oil

Miscellaneous

- almond milk (unsweetened)
- cocoa powder
- coconut milk
- coconut water
- decaf herbal tea
- frozen berries
- green tea
- low-sodium, fat-free chicken, beef, or vegetable stock
- protein powder
- (whey, soy, pea, or casein)
- rice milk (unsweetened)
- shredded coconut (unsweetened)
- sparkling water

Vegetables

- ancho chiles (dried)
- artichoke
- arugula
- asparagus
- avocado
- baby greens
- bamboo shoots
- beets
- bell peppers
- bok choy
- broccoli
- brussels sprouts
- cabbage
- carrots
- cauliflower
- celery
- collard greens
- cucumbers
- eggplant
- endive
- fennel
- garlic
- green beans
- jicama
- kale
- lettuce
- mushrooms
- olives
- onions
- parsnips
- peas
- pumpkin
- seaweed
- spaghetti squash
- spinach
- sprouts
- sweet potatoes
- swiss chard
- tomatoes
- turnips
- yams
- yellow squash
- zucchini

Fruits

apples	figs	papayas
apricots	kiwis	peaches
blackberries	lemons	pears
blueberries	limes	pomegranates
cantaloupe	mangoes	raspberries
coconuts	melons	strawberries
cranberries	nectarines	watermelons

Raw Nuts and Seeds

almonds	flaxseeds (whole and ground)	pistachios
Brazil nuts		pumpkin seeds
cashews	hazelnuts	sesame seeds
chestnuts	pecans	sunflower seeds
chia seeds	pine nuts	walnuts

Meat, Poultry, and Fish

anchovies	cod (black)	tuna (canned, in water)
beef (lean, grass-fed)	eggs	
	pork loin	tuna (fresh filets)
chicken breasts (skinless, boneless)	salmon (wild-caught)	turkey (ground, 99% fat-free)
chicken (organic, free-range)	sardines	turkey (whole)
	shrimp	
	tilapia	

Sweeteners

blackstrap molasses	pure maple syrup	raw honey
cacao nibs	pure palm sugar	xylitol
	stevia	

Superfoods

Some foods are simply better than others in terms of nutrient density. The super-foods listed below are not only cleanse-friendly, they're also nutritional powerhouses that will nourish your body at the cellular level, boost your immunity, and give you the energy to power through your workouts.

Leafy Greens

Calorie for calorie, these plants deliver more nutrients than just about any other food on the planet. Loaded with fiber; vitamins A, C, and K; folate; calcium; and tons of phytochemicals (plant-based chemicals)—leafy greens stock your body with the artillery needed to fight off potential killers like heart disease and cancer.

Leafy greens to try:

arugula

kale

mustard greens

spinach

swiss chard

Cruciferous Vegetables

Research suggests that cruciferous veggies have the ability to inhibit the growth of some types of cancer cells and even stop others by reducing the production of free radicals. They're also full of fiber and offer a great way to keep hunger at bay.

Cruciferous veggies to try:

bok choy

broccoli

brussels sprouts

cabbage

cauliflower

Avocado

Some people are afraid of avocados because they contain a lot of fat—and they do, but this is the kind of fat you *want* to include in your diet! Avocados contain oleic acid, lutein, folate, vitamin E, and lots of heart-healthy monosaturated fats. These work to protect against heart disease, cancer, and degenerative eye and brain diseases.

Great ways to use avocado:

spread on a sandwich in place of mayo

blend in a protein shake

chop into a salad

mash up in a dip (such as guacamole)

slice as a topping for eggs

Blueberries

This tiny fruit is packed with disease-fighting phytochemicals, flavinoids, and soluble fiber, all of which help to prevent diseases like cancer, diabetes, heart disease, stomach ulcers, and high blood pressure. They also help tame inflammation and can reduce "bad" (LDL) cholesterol.

Great ways to enjoy blueberries:

freeze and eat for dessert

blend in a smoothie

sprinkle on top of yogurt

eat with cereal

toss in a salad

Beans

Protein-rich beans contain tons of B vitamins, calcium, potassium, and folate. They also help raise levels of leptin, a hormone that curbs appetite and contributes to the maintenance of healthy brain, cell, and skin function.

Great ways to enjoy beans:

swap in for meat in tacos and wraps

serve as a side dish in place of potatoes

scoop on top of baked potatoes

pair with brown rice

blend into soups and sauces

Walnuts

These hearty nuts contain tons of omega-3 fatty acids, alpha-linolenic acid, mela-tonin, copper, manganese, and vitamin E, all of which help to protect your heart. Walnuts may also protect your brain and help slow the onset of Alzheimer's and Parkinson's disease.

Great ways to enjoy walnuts:

chop and add to cereal or oatmeal

toss into salads

blend into smoothies

add to trail mix

stir into sautés or stir-fries

Wild Salmon

Wild-caught salmon ranks high in nutrients and low in contaminants. Salmon is a rich source of protein, vitamin D, selenium, B vitamins, and those all-important omega-3 fatty acids. All these work in the body to protect against cancer, cardiovas-cular problems, macular degeneration, depression, and cognitive decline.

Great ways to prepare salmon:

baked

grilled

poached

broiled

pan-seared

Chocolate

Yes, you read that right! Dairy-free chocolate, in moderation, is a delicious treat that can help elevate mood, improve blood flow, and even lower blood pressure. It also helps reduce inflammation and LDL "bad" cholesterol, and is loaded with antioxidants, which can help prevent cell damage. But this doesn't give you license to pig out—keep your servings to one ounce a few times a week, and buy chocolate that is at least 70% cocoa.

Great ways to enjoy chocolate:

in a smoothie

as a dessert

in a molé sauce for chicken or beef

as a hot beverage with almond or soy milk

sprinkled on Greek yogurt

Chia Seeds

These little guys are the single richest source of plant-based omega-3 fatty acids you can buy. They're loaded with antioxidants, proteins, and minerals, plus soluble and insoluble fiber to help keep your digestion moving in the right direction. What's more, chia seeds swell to more than five times their weight in liquid, so adding a spoonful or two to meals helps you to feel full.

Great ways to enjoy chia seeds:

add to smoothies

stir into Greek yogurt

sprinkle over oatmeal or cereal

add to salads

use to crust fish

Chapter 14

The Recipes

Let thy food be medicine, thy medicine shall be thy food.

—HIPPOCRATES

I don't fancy myself a chef by any stretch of the imagination, so I got a little help from Dr. Frank Lipman, from various friends, and from my staff to come up with this collection of flavorful recipes, marinades, dressings, and desserts. They are all tasty, wholesome, and easy to prepare.

Breakfast

Smoothies are a great, easy way to get in a healthy breakfast. Here are three of my favorites. Simply mix all the ingredients in a blender, blend on high for 30–60 seconds, and serve immediately. Each of these makes one serving—a fast, nutritious breakfast.

Banana Berry Smoothie

1 small frozen banana, cut into
   chunks
1 c mixed frozen berries
1 scoop protein powder
½ c almond milk

½ c water
4 ice cubes

Pumpkin Pie Smoothie

1 scoop protein powder

½ c water

½ c unsweetened vanilla almond
   milk

1 c cooked or canned pumpkin

½ frozen banana

1 tsp vanilla extract

1 tsp coconut oil (optional)

4 ice cubes

dash of cinnamon

Chocoholic Protein Smoothie

1 scoop protein powder

½ c water

½ unsweetened vanilla almond
   milk

½ frozen banana

¼ avocado

1 tbsp cacao nibs

1 tsp honey

1 tbsp coconut oil

4 ice cubes

Want to get more veggies in your diet? Add kale or spinach to your morning shake. Don't be intimidated by the green smoothie—they taste great!

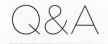

Q&A

QUESTION: What kind of protein powder should I use in my smoothie?

ANSWER: There are many kinds available, including soy, whey, casein, and even pea protein. Choosing a powder is a matter of personal taste as well as sensitivities. For instance, those with dairy intolerance should not have a product that contains casein, which is derived from milk, and some may also be sensitive to whey. Read the label carefully to make sure your product does not contain anything you cannot eat. Also check your product for added sugar.

Not a smoothie fan? Here are some other great breakfast ideas that taste great and give you plenty of energy.

Raw Muesli

8 oz uncooked rolled oats

1 c almond milk

1 tbsp unsweetened shredded coconut

2 tbsp chopped walnuts or almonds

2 tbsp ground flaxseeds

2 tbsp sesame seeds

2 tbsp pumpkin seeds

8 oz fresh berries

1 apple, peeled and grated

In a large bowl, mix together the oats, nut milk, shredded coconut, nuts, and seeds. Cover and place in fridge overnight. In the morning, add berries and grated apple and serve. Makes 4 servings.

Veggie-and-Rice Frittata

5 eggs

2 egg whites

2 tbsp fresh parsley, chopped

½ tsp salt, divided into two parts

½ tsp ground pepper, divided into two parts

¼ tsp ground nutmeg

2 tsp extra-virgin olive oil

½ c red onion, chopped

½ c green bell pepper, chopped

½ c mushrooms, chopped

½ c spinach, chopped

1 tbsp minced fresh rosemary (or 1 tsp dried)

1 ½ c brown rice, cooked

Preheat your broiler. Beat eggs and egg whites and combine with parsley, nutmeg, and half the salt and pepper. Heat the olive oil in a cast-iron skillet over medium heat. Add onion, salt, and pepper, and sauté until soft. Add rosemary and veggies and cook, stirring frequently until pan is almost dry of liquid (about 5–7 minutes). Reduce heat to medium-low and add the rice. Pour in the egg mixture and cook in the pan until partially set. Then place the pan in the oven under the broiler and cook until the top is browned. Let stand 5–10 minutes. Makes 4–6 servings.

Cinnamon Oatmeal

½ c whole oats, uncooked

1 scoop protein powder

1 tsp honey

¼ tsp flax or chia seeds

dash of cinnamon

Cook oats according to the instructions on the package. Add protein powder and honey and mix thoroughly. Top with cinnamon and seeds.

Lunch

A lot of people tend to have a variation on the same thing for lunch every day—a salad or a sandwich, something quick and on-the-go. But with a little planning and prep work you can make satisfying, tasty lunches to pack up and brown-bag during the workweek, or to simply take out of the fridge when you're busy at home. Remember to make large batches so that you get multiple servings out of one cooking session!

Spinach Salad with Shrimp and Mushrooms

4 c baby spinach leaves

1 avocado, peeled and sliced

1 c mushrooms, thinly sliced

2 tomatoes, sliced

½ c walnuts, chopped

12 oz cooked and peeled shrimp

Combine ingredients and toss with your favorite healthy dressing. Makes 2 servings.

Quinoa Tabouli Salad

1 c quinoa, cooked

1 c tomatoes, chopped

1 c cucumbers, chopped

½ c parsley, chopped

½ c mint, chopped

Lemon vinaigrette

¾ c extra-virgin olive oil

¼ c lemon juice

1 clove garlic, crushed

1 tsp salt

1 tsp mustard

ground black pepper to taste

Mix together ingredients for salad in a large bowl. Pour dressing ingredients into a shaker or glass jar and shake well until mixed. Drizzle a tablespoon of dressing onto one serving of salad. Makes 4 servings.

Stir-Fried Chicken and Vegetables

4 boneless, skinless organic chicken breasts, sliced

4 tbsp low-sodium soy sauce

1 tbsp mirin

2 tsp arrowroot

1 c low-sodium, low-fat chicken or vegetable stock

3 tbsp extra-virgin olive oil

1 large onion, sliced

2 garlic cloves, crushed

1 tbsp ginger, grated

3 carrots, sliced

2 celery stalks, sliced

2 c broccoli florets

1 c mushrooms, sliced

1 red bell pepper, sliced in strips

Red pepper flakes to taste (optional)

Marinate the chicken strips in 2 tbsp of the soy sauce and the mirin for 30 minutes, then drain. Mix arrowroot, remaining soy sauce, and chicken or vegetable stock, and set aside. Heat 1 tbsp olive oil in a skillet and stir-fry the chicken until cooked through. Remove and set aside. Heat remaining oil, then add the onion, garlic, ginger, and red pepper flakes (optional). Cook 2 minutes. Add carrots, celery, and broccoli, and cook until tender. Add remaining vegetables and cook for 2–3 minutes. Return chicken to the pan and add the sauce. Makes 4–6 servings.

Grass-Fed Beef Tacos

1 tbsp olive oil

1 tsp cumin

1 garlic clove, minced

6 oz grass-fed beefsteak, sliced

1 c green peppers, sliced

1 c red bell peppers, sliced

½ c onion, sliced

2 gluten-free tortillas, small

¼ c low-sodium salsa

¼ c shredded nondairy cheese

¼ c avocado, chopped

Sauté olive oil, cumin, and garlic for one minute. Add the beef and cook through. Add peppers and onion and cook until vegetables are soft. Spoon into gluten-free tortillas and top with salsa, avocado, and cheese. Makes 2 servings.

Turkey-Lettuce Sliders

1 lb lean or extra-lean ground
    turkey

1 whole egg, beaten

½ tsp garlic powder

¼ tsp salt

1 tbsp red onion, minced

1 tbsp fresh parsley, chopped

¼ tsp freshly ground black pepper

6 large lettuce leaves, torn in half

1 tsp olive oil

Mix together all ingredients but the lettuce leaves and olive oil. Form mixture into 10–12 small patties. Heat the olive oil in a skillet, moving it around so it covers the bottom. Cook patties 2–4 minutes, or until no longer pink in the center. Serve open faced on a lettuce leaf with your favorite healthy burger toppings. Makes 6 servings.

Dinner

Dinner is always a sticking point for women, especially if you have a family full of picky eaters! Here are some winning recipes that your whole gang will love. And they'll never know just how good for them these yummy meals are.

Simple Broccoli Soup

1 tbsp extra-virgin olive oil

1 medium onion, chopped

2 cloves fresh garlic, crushed

2 lbs broccoli, rinsed and chopped

1 tsp ground thyme

6–8 cups organic, low-sodium
   vegetable stock (how thick you

want the soup will dictate how
   much stock you use)

fresh chopped parsley, chives,
   or dill

salt and freshly ground pepper
   (to taste)

In a large pot, heat the oil and sauté the onion and garlic until onion is soft and translucent. Add the remaining ingredients and bring to a boil. Cover, reduce heat, and simmer until the broccoli is tender, about 40 minutes. Transfer the soup to a blender and purée until smooth (or until it reaches your desired texture). Pour into bowls and garnish with fresh parsley, chives, or dill. Makes 6–8 servings.

Roasted Herbed Tilapia Filets

4 tilapia filets

juice of 1 large lemon

1 clove garlic, crushed

¼ c fresh oregano, chopped

¼ c fresh basil, chopped

¼ c fresh parsley, chopped

1 tsp extra-virgin olive oil

salt and pepper (to taste)

lemon wedges (optional)

Preheat oven to 375°. Mix together the herbs, garlic, and olive oil and set aside. Squeeze lemon juice over fish filets, then spread the herb mixture evenly over the fish. Roast fish in the oven until cooked through, about 12–15 minutes. Serve with lemon wedges if desired. Makes 4 servings.

Vegetable Curry

1 onion, chopped

2 cloves garlic, crushed

2 tbsp extra-virgin olive oil

½–1 tsp curry powder (depending on your preference)

1 tsp cumin

½ tsp coriander

¼ tsp cinnamon

¼ tsp ground ginger

¼ tsp turmeric

½ tsp salt

½ butternut squash, peeled and cut into small cubes

¾ c water

1 large sweet potato, peeled and cubed

½ cauliflower, cut into florets

¾ c frozen organic peas

½ tsp garam masala

cilantro (optional)

To a medium-sized pot add the olive oil, onion, and garlic and sauté over medium heat until the onions are soft and translucent. Add the spices and salt and cook for an additional 2–3 minutes. Add the butternut squash and sweet potato and sauté about 10 minutes, stirring occasionally and adding water as needed to prevent sticking. Add the rest of the water and scrape all the spices up from the bottom of the pot. Add cauliflower and peas. Cover and cook until the vegetables are tender, about 10–15 minutes. Just before serving, add garam masala and stir through. Sprinkle with cilantro if desired. Makes 4 servings.

Roasted Mediterranean Vegetables

1 yellow pepper

1 red pepper,

4 oz cherry tomatoes

1 eggplant

2 cloves garlic

A few sprigs of rosemary and oregano

2 tbsp olive oil

Peheat the oven to 400°. Prepare the vegetables and place in a large roasting pan.

Place the herbs between the vegetables and sprinkle with the crushed garlic. Drizzle over the oil and turn the vegetables gently so they are coated in a little olive oil.

Roast in the oven for 30-40 minutes or until the vegetables are tender. Makes 4 servings.

Spicy Chicken

4 skinless boneless organic chicken
    breasts
¼ c red wine vinegar
¼ c extra-virgin olive oil
½ tsp freshly ground black pepper

1 tsp dried oregano
½ tsp crushed red pepper
1 clove garlic, crushed
½ tsp paprika
1 tsp salt

In a small bowl, whisk together all ingredients—except for the chicken—to create a marinade. Place the chicken in a casserole dish and pour the marinade over chicken. Cover and place in the fridge at least one hour or overnight. When ready to cook the chicken, place each breast on a lightly oiled grill pan or skillet over medium-high heat. Cook each side for approximately five minutes, or until cooked through. Serve over brown rice with a side of steamed veggies. Makes 4 servings.

Wild-Caught Sesame Salmon

4 wild-caught salmon filets (6 oz
    each)
4 tbsp low-sodium soy sauce
2 tbsp rice vinegar
2 tbsp sesame oil

1 tbsp agave nectar (or stevia)
2 tbsp black sesame seeds
2 tbsp white sesame seeds
½ tsp salt
1 lemon, sliced into wedges

In a small bowl, whisk together the soy sauce, vinegar, sesame oil, and agave nectar (or stevia) to make a marinade. Place the filets into a casserole dish and pour the marinade over the fish. Marinate for about 15 minutes.

Preheat oven to 400°. Place filets into a baking dish, skin side down. Mix together seeds and salt, and sprinkle over filets, pressing mixture firmly into fish so it adheres. Place into the oven and bake for about 12–15 minutes, or until cooked through. Serve with lemon wedges. Makes 4 servings.

Quick Veggie Sides

Side of Roasted Vegetables

(You can use any seasonal vegetables)

450 g pumpkin,

2 carrots, peeled and halved

4 parsnips, peeled and quartered

1 large sweet potato, peeled and
   cut into chunks

A few sprigs rosemary

2 garlic cloves, crushed

Salt and pepper

2 tbsp olive oil

Preheat oven to 400°. Prepare the vegetables and place in a large roasting pan.

Place the herbs between the vegetables and sprinkle with the crushed garlic, salt, and pepper. Drizzle the oil and turn the vegetables gently so they are coated in oil.

Roast in the oven for 30–40 minutes or until the vegetables are tender. Makes 4 servings.

Spicy Spinach and Mushrooms

1 tbsp extra-virgin olive oil

1 medium onion, chopped

1 clove garlic, crushed

1 tsp fresh ginger, grated

1 tsp chili powder

½ lb mushrooms, thinly sliced

1 lb spinach, washed (or bagged
   organic baby spinach)

salt (to taste)

Heat the oil in a large skillet. Add onion and garlic and stir-fry until browned. Add the spices and stir-fry for about one minute. Add mushrooms and salt. When the mushrooms have softened, add the spinach and cook until the spinach has wilted. Makes 4 servings.

Parsnip and Sweet Potato "Fries"

2 large parsnips, peeled and sliced
   longways
1 large sweet potato, sliced into
   strips

olive oil
sea salt

Preheat oven to 400°. Place parsnip and sweet potato slices in a zip-top bag. Add salt, pepper, and olive oil. Shake until coated. Spread onto a baking sheet in a single layer. Bake until tender (45–60 minutes), turning several times to cook evenly. Makes 4 servings.

Snacks

Snacks don't need to be complicated, but they do need to be healthy. Here are some ideas for snacks that are easy to make and taste great. And remember: you can always eat half of a meal serving as a snack!

- carrots or celery with about ¼ cup hummus
- 1 apple cut into slices, with 1 tbsp almond butter for dipping
- ¼ cup raw nuts and a banana
- ½ cup quinoa tabouli salad with small handful of cashews
- 1 cup low-fat Greek yogurt with ¼ cup berries
- 1 oz canned tuna with about 10 rice crackers
- 1 hard-boiled egg and a piece of whole fruit
- a few rice crackers topped with 2 slices avocado and 2 oz turkey breast

Veggies

I love to eat my veggies raw, but sometimes I also crave them piping hot, especially in the winter. What's better than a bowl of roasted Brussels sprouts or some sautéed kale with a side of brown rice? Yum. The tricky thing when it comes to cooking veggies is to make sure you don't overcook them. Overcooking not only impacts flavor, it also decreases the nutritional value. Here are a few tips:

Steaming

Steaming vegetables locks in more of the nutritive vitamins and minerals than boiling. Vegetable steamers are fairly cheap and can also be used to prepare other foods like rice and fish. Steamer baskets—which you place in a pot of boiling water to create an instant steamer—are another easy and inexpensive option.

Sautéing

When you sauté veggies you want to make sure you add just a little olive oil, and that your pan is super hot. Slice the vegetables thinly so that they cook quickly. Keep an eye on the color of your veggies as they cook—bright greens like broccoli, spinach, and kale can quickly turn dark green, at which point you've lost flavor and nutrients. Sauté veggies until just tender, then remove from heat.

Roasting

Roasting is a great option for heartier veggies such as root vegetables. Slice your vegetables into chunks and toss them with a little olive oil, just enough to coat them. Spread the vegetables in a single layer in a roasting pan. Bake at 400° until tender, usually around 20–45 minutes, depending on the type of vegetable.

Treats

As you know, I allow myself a small treat every day! But these treats are so healthy I don't know if I'd really consider them cheating. Try whipping up one of these easy recipes when your sweet tooth simply won't quiet down.

Walnut-Date Balls

2 c walnuts

1 c dates, pitted

3 tbsp fresh lemon juice

1/3 c unsweetened coconut, shredded

Chop the nuts in a food processor. Add the dates and lemon juice. Pulse until well blended and the mixture starts to stick together. Form into small balls and roll into shredded coconut. Place in fridge to harden for 30 minutes before eating.

Chocolate Fudge

16-oz jar nut butter (almond or cashew)

¼ c unsweetened cocoa powder

½ c agave syrup

2 tbsp vanilla extract

1 tsp sea salt

Mix all ingredients, minus the sea salt, in a food processor. Line an 8 x 8 cake pan with parchment paper. Spoon the mixture into the pan and pat down. Sprinkle with sea salt. Cover tightly with foil and place in freezer for about 1 hour. Remove from freezer and cut into small squares and serve immediately. Keep in the freezer to prevent fudge from turning soft and mushy. Makes about 30 squares.

Banana-Strawberry Sorbet

1 banana, frozen and cut into
    chunks
1 c frozen strawberries

½ tsp vanilla extract
1 tsp agave syrup

In a food processor, combine all the ingredients and blend until smooth and creamy. Serve immediately or transfer to an airtight container and refreeze for later. Makes 2 servings.

Rubs, Sauces, Dressings, and Marinades

Sometimes healthy food suffers from a lack of flavor: simple steamed or poached veggies and proteins can be a little bland, and I am a girl who likes to have her palate wowed. These simple rubs, sauces, dressings, and marinades can be made in advance and are a great way to create layers of unique flavor without adding lots of sodium.

All-Purpose Rub

This rub is perfect for grilling chicken—the herbs give a nice fresh balance to the smokiness and char of the grill. You could also use this mix for cooking flaky white fish, such as tilapia fillets.

1 tsp garlic powder
1 tsp ground thyme
3 tsp dried rosemary

3 tsp dried oregano
1 tsp salt
1 tsp fresh ground pepper

Indian Spice Rub

Use Indian spice–rubbed chicken in wraps, salads, or as a dinner entrée, served with fresh roasted vegetables and brown rice.

1 tsp cumin

1 tsp coriander

1 tsp turmeric

1 tsp garam masala

½ tsp garlic powder

½ tsp ginger powder

pinch of cayenne pepper

Lemon and Olive Oil Marinade

Whisk this quick marinade together, pour over chicken, and allow it to marinate overnight. Pan-fry marinated chicken and toss into salads, sandwiches, or serve as an entrée.

¾ c extra-virgin olive oil

juice of 2 large lemons

1 tbsp fresh chopped parsley

1 tsp salt

4 cloves garlic, crushed

1 tsp mustard powder

1 tsp dried oregano

1 tsp ground black pepper

Mustard-and-Rosemary Marinade

This flavorful marinade is delicious on salmon. Coat the skinless side of a salmon filet with marinade. Set aside for 10 minutes. Pan-fry until cooked through, turning once.

2 tbsp whole-grain mustard

1 tbsp extra-virgin olive oil

juice of 1 large lemon

1 clove garlic, crushed

1 tbsp fresh rosemary, chopped

salt and pepper to taste

Tandoori Marinade

This sweet and spicy marinade is the perfect accompaniment to chicken, lamb, or salmon. Marinate meat overnight—but in the case of salmon, only for about 10 minutes—and pour off excess marinade. Bake at 350°, turning and basting it half-way through with the excess marinade.

¾ c plain yogurt

4 cloves garlic, crushed

1 tsp garlic powder

2 tsp fresh ginger, grated

1 tsp salt

½ tsp cumin

½ tsp cayenne pepper

2 tsp coriander

1 tbsp paprika

½ tsp turmeric

½ tsp cinnamon

2 tbsp lemon juice

Balsamic Vinaigrette

⅔ c extra virgin olive oil

⅓ c balsamic vinegar

1 clove garlic, crushed

1 tsp Dijon mustard

1 tsp raw honey

pinch of salt

Put all ingredients into a small bowl and whisk together. Makes 1 cup of dressing, approximately 16 tablespoons (8–16 servings).

Wheat-Free Soy Vinaigrette

1 tbsp wheat-free soy sauce or
   tamari

½ c extra-virgin olive oil

¼ c apple cider vinegar (or juice of
   2 limes)

1 tsp raw honey

1 small red chili, seeded and finely
   chopped (or dash of red pepper
   flakes)

1 tbsp sesame oil

Put all ingredients into a small bowl and whisk together. Makes 1 cup of dressing, approximately 16 tablespoons (8–16 servings).

Tomato Puttanesca Sauce

This fresh, spicy sauce is incredible over gluten-free pasta, roasted chicken, and even white fish. Try doubling the recipe and freezing some for another time!

2 tbsp extra-virgin olive oil

2 cloves garlic, crushed

2 c chopped tomatoes (or 1 can, low-sodium, drained)

½ c kalamata olives, pitted and chopped

½ c capers, rinsed and drained

red pepper flakes (optional)

Heat the oil and add the garlic, cooking for 1 minute. Add tomatoes and red pepper flakes and cook for 10 minutes, stirring occasionally. Add olives and capers and cook for 2 minutes. Makes 1 cup of sauce, approximately 2 servings.

Perfect Pesto

Pesto is the perfect complement to chicken and mild-flavored fish like tilapia. It also makes a great sauce for healthy carbohydrates such as gluten-free pasta and brown rice. Because the ingredients pack a punch of flavor, a little pesto goes a long way, so one batch will last you a while. Pesto should be stored in the fridge to stay fresh.

2 c fresh basil leaves

2 cloves garlic

¼ c pine nuts

⅔ c extra-virgin olive oil

salt and pepper (to taste)

Combine basil, garlic, and pine nuts in a food processor and pulse until coarsely chopped. Add olive oil and blend until smooth. Season with salt and pepper. Makes about 1 cup of pesto, or 16 one-tablespoon servings.

Molé Sauce

This sauce is rich, savory, and hearty, with a lovely smoky flavor that is unlike anything else. Marinate meats such as turkey, chicken, and pork overnight to absorb the full spectrum of flavors.

3 white onions, quartered

4 plum tomatoes, quartered

3 cloves garlic, peeled

2 banana peppers

3 ancho chiles, dried

1 tsp chili powder

1 tsp unsweetened cocoa powder

2 c chicken or vegetable stock

1 lime, juiced and zested

Set the oven to broil. Combine all veggies except the ancho chiles and spread evenly on a sheet pan. Broil veggies on the top rack, stirring frequently, until tomatoes begin to bubble. Remove and cool. In a small bowl, place the chiles and cover with boiling water. Allow to steep for 10 minutes. Remove chiles and trim stems. Put chiles and veggies in a food processor and blend until smooth. Put the purée in a saucepan and add the remaining spices (except the lime and zest). Cook on medium heat for 20–30 minutes. Top with lime juice and zest.

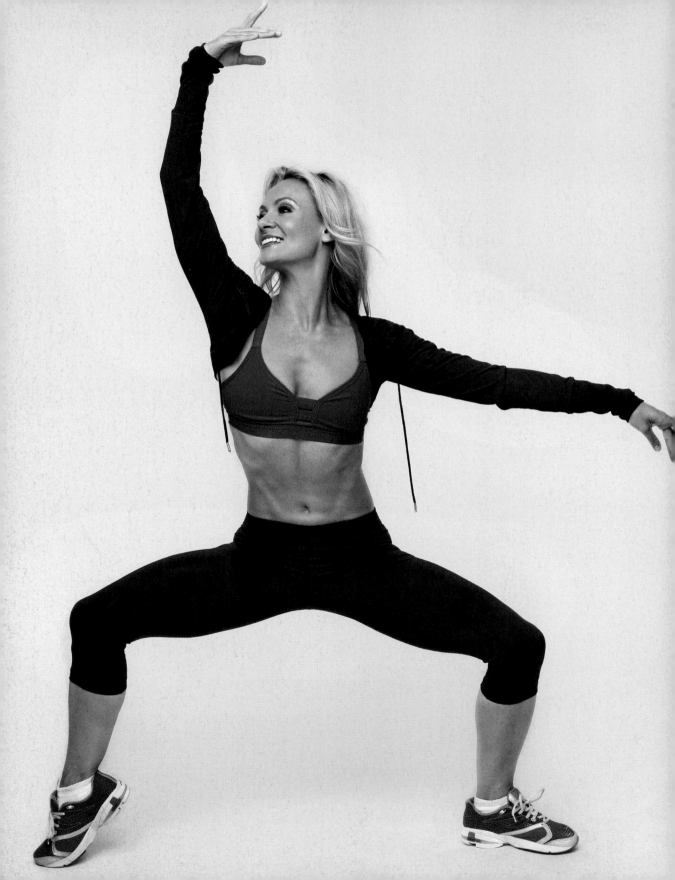

The
Performance

Chapter 15
Blocking the Steps

You dance love, and you dance joy, and you dance dreams.
And I know if I can make you smile by jumping over a couple
of couches or running through a rainstorm, then I'll be very
glad to be a song and dance man.

—GENE KELLY

Now that you've got the nuts and bolts of your workouts, it's time to put everything together. We all lead busy lives, but making time to exercise is essential.

Duration

You may be wondering exactly how long your workouts will take. Here's how it breaks down: each time you exercise you're going to do both a Strength and a Cardio work-out, plus your Mirror Minutes, a warm-up, and a cool-down/stretch. This comes to approximately 40–60 minutes, total.

This number will vary somewhat from person to person, since everyone is starting at a different level and will spend varying amounts of time warming up, recovering between moves, and stretching afterward. Regardless, I always suggest dedicating a full hour to your workout, even if you don't use that entire hour. Giving yourself that time will ensure you'll never be rushed or tempted to skip parts of your session in an effort to finish within a shorter time frame. If it makes it easier to fit into your schedule, you can do 30 minutes in the morning and 30 minutes in the evening—whatever will get you to stick to your plan!

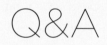

QUESTION: I only have 20 minutes to work out. Which part of the workout should I do and which should I skip, the Strength or the Cardio?

ANSWER: Both are equally important so I don't recommend skipping either one. Remember: the Strength workouts build muscle and tone up your body from head to toe, while the Cardio workouts burn fat and increase your energy level. Do shorter versions of both, with accelerated warm-ups and stretches, for a complete workout session.

Approximate Workout Times (Strength and Cardio Combined)

Level I: Corps de Ballet	30 minutes
Level II: Soloist	45 minutes
Level III: Principal	60 minutes

Frequency

How often you work out will depend on your current fitness level. Those who are just starting out will need more time between sessions to recover, while those at a higher fitness level can work out more frequently. Here are a few sample workout weeks for each of the three Levels of the BBS program:

Level I: Corps de Ballet

Level I exercisers should be working out at least three days a week. Allow yourself about a day in between sessions to rest and recover properly. If you need more than one day to recover in the beginning, give yourself that time. Perhaps stretch and work on your flexibility on that day instead of doing a workout: warm up a little by walking around the block or marching in place for 5–10 minutes, then do the stretching routine outlined on page 123. This will help improve your range of motion and decrease your soreness, so you can be ready to work out again sooner.

Sample Level I: Corps de Ballet Workout Schedule

MONDAY	TUESDAY	WEDNESDAY	THURSDAY	FRIDAY	SATURDAY	SUNDAY
BBS workout	Rest	BBS workout	Rest	BBS workout	Rest	Rest

Level II: Soloist

Level II exercisers, you should be working out at least 4 days a week. I suggest spacing your rest days out during the week, taking them every few days, or when you feel overly sore or tired. On the other hand, if you're feeling good, get in that extra workout on your fifth day! I always like to take advantage of days when I am filled with pep to get a little more exercise.

Sample Level II: Soloist Workout Schedule

MONDAY	TUESDAY	WEDNESDAY	THURSDAY	FRIDAY	SATURDAY	SUNDAY
BBS workout	BBS workout	Rest	BBS workout	Rest	BBS workout	Rest or optional BBS workout

Level III: Principal

Level III, you should be working out 5–6 days per week, with 1–2 days of rest. It's very important to take days off, no matter how advanced you are. It's those days off where your body recovers from the work you've been giving it, and taking that time helps prevent injury and can even reset your mind so you're eager to resume your workout the next day! I know that if I take a few days off from the gym, I can't wait to get back after a good solid rest. I suggest spacing your rest days out during the week to give your body a break more than once.

Sample Level III: Principal Workout Schedule

MONDAY	TUESDAY	WEDNESDAY	THURSDAY	FRIDAY	SATURDAY	SUNDAY
BBS workout	BBS workout	BBS workout	Rest	BBS workout	BBS workout	Rest or BBS workout

Forward Thinking

I recommend planning your workouts at least a week in advance, scheduling them into your calendar like any other time commitment, such as a work meeting or a doctor's visit. Because they are just as important.

Now get out your planner or pull up your scheduling app and look at your week ahead. What events do you have coming up? Are you in town or are you traveling? Are there family functions to consider, or any social events you need to work around? Write all these things into your schedule, then take a realistic look at your day-to-day life. Where will a workout fit in? It might not be apparent at first, but if you look hard enough, you will find the time. If it seems impossible, then move some things around and *make* the time. Remember: this is about you and your mental and physical health. Nothing is more important than that! Planning your workouts into your weekly routine solidifies your resolve and acts as a reminder of your commitment to yourself and your goals.

And once you write your workouts in your schedule, stick to them. Don't bump them off and replace them with something else, or let anyone talk you out of doing them in favor of other things during that time. This time is for you, and it is essential to your mental and physical health.

Here are some ideas to help you find or make the time to exercise:

- Get up 30 minutes earlier each day and do at least half of your workout.
- Do several 10–20-minute mini-workouts on days when you're super busy.
- Use your lunch hour to exercise.
- Do your workout while your kids are in sports or afterschool activities.
- Instead of meeting up with your girlfriends for happy hour, meet up for a workout.
- Exercise during your "TV time."

Of course, there will be times when your lovely little plan does not work—your car breaks down, work runs into lunch, your alarm doesn't go off. Life is full of surprises, and something may come up that prevents you from sticking to your schedule and you miss a workout. Relax—if you found the time once, you can find it again! Use that missed workout as one of your rest days and regroup. Take a deep breath, then look at your schedule once more and see where you can fit in a new workout. I know you can do it!

Q&A

QUESTION: I like the idea of 10-minute workouts, but seriously, how can working out for 10 minutes possibly be worth it?

ANSWER: There's actually a lot of research that validates the effectiveness of these mini-workouts, so don't discount them! Moving your body and getting your heart rate up boosts metabolism and sparks fat burning while improving blood flow to your muscles and your brain. Now imagine doing that three times a day! Besides, a 10-minute workout is better than no workout at all.

Here's a great 10-minute workout that will blast fat fast. Do each move for one minute:

1. Jump Rope
2. Band Curlers
3. Double Curl and Reach
4. Jump rope
5. Pony Kick
6. Ball-abesque
7. Froggy
8. Hip Slimmer II
9. Double Towel Slider
10. Window Washer

No Excuses

I have some of the busiest clients on the planet! If they can find the time to work out, so can you. In fact, I train some of my celebrity clients on set, while they're filming! In between takes, we squeeze in 10-minute workouts so that they can get in their exercise and have the strength and stamina they need to perform physically demanding roles.

My client Anne Hathaway also trains while filming. When she is short on time (some days she'll shoot for 12 hours straight!), she does this workout using wrist weights:

MOVE	REPS
Swan Arms	20
Sliders	20
Breaststroke	20
Great Guns	20, each arm
Glute Burnout	20–30, each leg
Froggy	20–30
Single Knee drop	20, each leg
Towel Slider	20, each leg

Progressing

As you exercise and become more fit, you might notice that things that were once challenging have become easier, and a routine that once had you gasping for air is now less of an oxygen-suck. Isn't that an amazing feeling? It means you're becoming healthier, and stronger, and gaining endurance. It means your muscles are growing and your heart and lungs working more efficiently. It means that oxygen is flowing through your body, giving you energy and delivering nutrients to all of your cells. And it means that your brain is firing on all cylinders and allowing you to feel happy, sharp, and clear-minded.

The BBS program is created to evolve with you as you reach new fitness goals and become stronger, faster, and better. Here are a few ways to keep yourself challenged as you progress:

- CHANGE YOUR LEVEL, even if it means moving from a higher one to a lower one. Your body thrives on variety, and the more challenges you can give it, the better. All my workouts are fun and demanding in different ways, so even if you're a Level III exerciser, you can find new and stimulating things to do in Level I. And of course, if you've been working in Level I or II, try moving to Level II or III.
- INCREASE THE RESISTANCE. Choose a heavier dumbbell or thicker resistance band to challenge your muscles in the Strength workouts. I don't recommend using dumbbells that are heavier than 3–5 pounds, but for those who have started with no weights or with 1–2 pounders, there is room to grow.
- DECREASE THE REST INTERVAL. Shortening the time you spend resting and recovering between Strength moves will push your body to work harder, increasing your heart rate and calorie burn. Try clipping 15–30 seconds off your current rest interval and see how you feel.
- ADD ANOTHER WORKOUT TO YOUR WEEK. In Levels I and II, you have room to grow with your schedule, and adding another workout to your week could be just the challenge you need to move forward and keep progressing.
- ADD MORE REPS. For each strength move, I've given you a suggested rep range to shoot for, so if you've been working in the lower part of that range, add a few more reps and see what happens. If you've already maxed out of

that range, that's totally fine—just do more reps! The table is only a guideline; and, truthfully, in my classes we sometimes get near the 100-rep range for certain moves, depending on the music and the energy in the room!

- ADD MORE TIME. The Cardio workouts are done to music, so toss a few more songs onto your playlist to make the sessions longer. And if you're adding more reps to your Strength workout, you'll naturally add more time to your session.

- INCREASE THE DRAMA. Dance is all about big, bold motions, and the more you can infuse drama into your Cardio workout, the more muscles you'll use and the higher your heart rate will climb!

Chapter 16
Becoming
the Dance

Practice is a means of inviting the perfection desired.

—MARTHA GRAHAM

One of the most important lessons I want you to take away from this book is that no exercise or nutrition plan will work over the long term if you don't make it part of your overall lifestyle. Creating healthy habits is the only way to ensure sustainable weight loss and lifelong health. At the end of these eight weeks, your new eating and exercise regimen will, hopefully, have become second nature—and the changes you'll experience in your mind and body will prove so motivating that you'll want to keep going full speed ahead!

That said, we all face challenges to our goals; life throws curveballs every day, and you've got to be prepared. Here are a few tools to help you navigate these rough spots so you can recover your stride and get back onto your path with minimal stress.

The Social Function

Going out and being social at parties is a fantastic part of life, but it can wreak havoc with your wellness program. It's a slippery slope, since you don't want to offend your host by refusing to eat their carefully prepared meal or finger tasties, but you also don't want to derail your resolve in favor of being polite. It's easy to overeat or indulge in foods you normally wouldn't eat when you're away from home and around friends and relatives. But there are ways you can be social and enjoy yourself without falling off the bandwagon!

- NEVER GO HUNGRY. If you arrive at a dinner or a party and you're famished, it's going to be very hard to resist those warm fresh rolls or delectable hors d'oeuvres! Have a nutritious snack about an hour beforehand that includes a protein and some fiber to fill you up. That way you can taste a few nibbles, without needing to make a whole meal of them.

- THINK BEFORE YOU DRINK. Alcohol has a lot of calories, so if you're going to indulge, choose your drink with care. Pick wine over drinks mixed with fruit juice and sugar, and just say no to specialty cocktails. Also, for every cocktail you drink, have at least one full glass of water. This will help slow your drinking pace while counteracting the dehydrating effect of alcohol on your system.

- FORGET THE FINGER FOODS. Typically, the appetizers passed around at parties are fried, laden with cheese, or wrapped in puff pastry—all total fat bombs! Choose skewered meats or veggie apps when possible, and nibble them slowly.

- SWAP PLATES. When in a buffet line, use a dinner plate for your salad and a salad plate for your dinner. It's difficult to overeat when you can't fit much on your plate!

- RESIGN AS A MEMBER OF THE "CLEAN PLATE CLUB." Even though your mother probably required you to finish everything on your plate—I know mine did—you are under no obligation to do so anymore! In fact, I discourage this habit, especially when you're at a function. For instance, if you choose a food at a buffet or party, or are served something and it isn't absolutely amazing, don't finish it. A treat is one thing, but there's no need to eat something you don't absolutely love!

- **SHARE AND SHARE ALIKE.** If your sweet tooth is screaming to be fed, go ahead and have dessert. You are allowed one day off with the BBS plan, so choose something you're craving and savor every bite. Better yet, share a treat with several other people. And remember: you are not obligated to finish it if it isn't fantastic.

Dining Out

Many of my clients frequent restaurants for work-related meals as well as for social time, and chances are if you're going to slip up in your plan, it will happen while you're dining out. Of course you could use a special night out as your "cheat" meal for the week and not worry about it. But if that "one night" turns into two or three or four, then you'll need to remember these tips on dining out healthfully:

- **LOOK UP THE RESTAURANT MENU ONLINE.** This way you'll know what you're in for, and how you might make accommodations to fit your plan.
- **GO GREEN.** Have a salad or a plate of fresh veggies as an appetizer, or fill half your dinner plate with greens and veggies and eat them first before you dig into your meal. Not only will you get a big blast of nutrients from the veggies, you'll also fill yourself up significantly, decreasing your chances of eating foods you'll want to avoid.
- **ASK FOR SAUCES AND DRESSINGS ON THE SIDE.** That way *you* control how much of it is added to your meal, not the chef.
- **BE SPECIFIC.** Order meats broiled, baked, or grilled, and have vegetables prepared steamed or raw whenever possible. Also, ask that all your food be prepared with little or no butter. A lot of people have dairy allergies these days, so this is not an uncommon request.
- **PASS THE BREAD.** If bread arrives at your table, pass it down to the other end. If the entire table is amenable, ask the server not to bring any at all.
- **FILL UP ON SOUP.** Choose dairy-free soups with vegetable, chicken, or tomato bases. Pair a bowl of soup with a salad or healthy appetizer for a filling meal.

Mental Recovery

Most people feel guilty or even angry with themselves when they stray from their plan, but missing one workout or eating one cookie is not the end of the world; it happens. Remember the negative/positive self-talk we addressed in Chapter 2? This can be a really good tool to use when you're feeling guilty about your misstep. Write out how you're feeling about what happened, then flip it to a positive perspective. For instance, the negative:

"I am so mad I missed my workout because of a business meeting!"
"Why could I not control myself at that brunch buffet?!"
"I let my friend talk me into going out for drinks instead of doing my workout. I am spineless!"

Now the positive:

"I got so much done at work tonight that I'll be able to exercise longer tomorrow!"
"Brunch was delicious. I will use that as my cheat meal for the week!"
"I was glad to spend some quality time with my friends. I needed it after a long week. Tomorrow I will get up 30 minutes earlier and do the workout I missed."

See how that works? In each instance this person didn't let guilt steamroll her, but rather made a plan of action to incorporate and embrace the happenings in her life and make them work *for* her, rather than against her. Remember: take it all in stride and get back on track as soon as possible, without regrets.

Get Your Zzzzzs

One way to ensure success is to make sure you're getting enough rest. And by rest, I don't mean lounging around, watching TV . . . I mean getting restorative, repairing, refreshing sleep. And plenty of it.

Research suggests that getting enough sleep is a cornerstone of maintaining a healthy weight. Numerous studies have shown that people who get at least seven hours of sleep per night have a lower body-fat percentage than those who get less rest. Sleep is also a time when your body produces the hormones that control appetite, such as leptin (an appetite suppressant) and grehlin (an appetite stimulant); sleep loss reduces the production of leptin while elevating the levels of grehlin. Translation: you feel you're "starving" when you get up, even if you're not in dire need of food. This can lead to overeating or poor food choices later in the day.

Being drowsy can also affect your decision-making when it comes to nutrition: you'll be searching for a quick-energy boost and will most probably reach for something easy that's sweet or salty, like cookies or chips, as well as a caffeinated beverage (or two, or three . . .). Sleep deprivation also causes an increase in cortisol, the nasty little hormone that makes you store body fat, and which is not something you want to have hanging out in your cells in excess. So by all means, sleep away! Try your best to get at least 8 hours of uninterrupted sleep per night. Go to bed at a decent hour and DVR the *Late Show* to watch over the weekend instead.

Q&A

QUESTION: How do I stick to my program during the holidays? There are so many parties and functions that I barely have time to do anything else.

ANSWER: The holidays are a time to celebrate with friends and family, so don't worry so much about losing weight during this time, but focus instead on maintaining your current weight and level of fitness. That way you can enjoy yourself and be social. Try your best to limit your treats and nibbles; schedule exercise into your day like you do in any given week; and don't let anyone talk you out of your workouts. Holidays are not only filled with treats, but also with stress—working out is a guaranteed stress relief!

QUESTION: I travel a lot. How can I take the BBS program with me and fit it into my away-from-home schedule?

ANSWER: Lots of my clients are busy women who travel frequently. Fortunately, you don't need much in the way of equipment to do these workouts! Just pack your resistance band, jump rope, this book, and your MP3 player and you're good to go. Clear out a space in your hotel room, just like you'd do at home, and go for it. Exercise before your work meetings to energize your body and your brain, or train after your meetings to destress and unwind. The stretching routine is also great to do post-flight to dekink yourself after sitting in an airplane.

Chapter 17
Performance of a Lifetime

Dance for yourself. If someone understands, good. If not, no matter. Go right on doing what interests you, and do it until it stops interesting you.

—LOUIS HORST

Even the most dedicated exerciser will feel less than motivated at times. The trick is not to let it get you down. Some people have the ability to just flip a switch in their mind and never deviate from their course; but for most people—including me!—it's tougher than that.

Motivation comes in different forms for different people, and there are lots of different ways to give yourself a little kick in the booty when you're feeling less than inspired to continue your program. Check out some of these suggestions, and use them when you feel like you need a little inspiration.

Revisit Your Goals

Sometimes a reminder of what you want to accomplish is all it takes to reenergize your motivation. Back in Chapter 4 we discussed goal setting and I asked you to choose a goal to reach by the end of this program and write it down. Hopefully you did so, and have been working hard to reach it! If you haven't already, write down your end goal on a piece of paper and put it where you can see it every day. Read and reflect on this goal whenever you feel like you need a little push to get you moving forward again. Personally, I like to visualize the outcome of how I will look and feel once I reach my goal: for instance, I picture my pants fitting better, my body looking amazing, and my energy level going through the roof!

Also, make those mini-goals we talked about before—things that you can reach easily on a weekly or even daily basis for extra motivation. Vow to drink more water today, or do a few more reps in your strength workout. Accomplishing these smaller goals is satisfying and empowering.

Tune Up

Nothing gets me going more than a new playlist! I love to change my music every other week or so and create new playlists to keep me motivated and eager to do my workouts. Out of ideas? Try making theme playlists like "Throwback 80s," "Friday Night Music," or "Michael Jackson Dance Party." And of course, you can always buy new tunes to put a little more spark in your step!

Check It Off

I don't know about you, but I like making lists, and checking things off of them makes me feel like I've accomplished something in my day. Even if you're not a list maker, try this technique: write out your to-dos for the day, including your workouts, your errands, your meals, and your work events—anything and everything that is going to happen that day. Once you complete the task or the workout, put a big check next to it, or cross it out. Trust me, it is an awesome feeling.

Girlfriend Workout

Nothing beats spending time with your girlfriends, and working out is no exception! I highly recommend buddying up with a friend or two and having a real Girlfriend Workout. Tons of research suggests that exercising with a friend increases adherence to a program, since workout partners provide motivation as well as accountability. Plus, you both get into shape and have fun doing it!

Movies as Motivation

Need a little visual inspiration? Here are some of my favorite dance movies of all time.

TOP HAT (1935): This movie was written expressly for Fred Astaire and Ginger Rogers, the smoothest duo ever to hit the ballroom stage (or screen).

SINGIN' IN THE RAIN (1952): Gene Kelly inspires thousands to ruin their shoes by dancing in puddles!

SATURDAY NIGHT FEVER (1977): Love disco or hate it, there are some great dance scenes in here. Plus, you get to see a young John Travolta in some seriously tight pants!

THE TURNING POINT (1977): My all-time idol Mikhail Baryshnikov stars with Shirley MacLaine and Anne Bancroft in a drama set in the realm of ballet.

FAME (1980): Students at New York's High School of Performing Arts come of age and dance through the streets of the city—and on top of taxicabs.

FLASHDANCE (1983): A welder/exotic dancer wants to get into ballet school—and gets doused in that infamous water scene.

FOOTLOOSE (1984): Kevin Bacon brings dance and music back to a sleepy farm community and wakes up the whole town in the process.

WHITE NIGHTS (1985): Crazy incredible tap dancer Gregory Hines stars alongside Baryshnikov. Must-see scene: the dance battle where Baryshnikov does eleven pirouettes like it was nothing!

A CHORUS LINE (1985): A movie inspired by the long-running Broadway musical. You'll be singing "One" for days afterward!

DIRTY DANCING (1987): Patrick Swayze proves that no one should put Baby in a corner when he leads Jennifer Grey through a sultry duet and into infamy.

STRICTLY BALLROOM (1992): A male ballroom dancer refuses to stick to the rules of the sport and tries out a new style of dance. Love, love, *love* the costumes and hairdos in this movie!

BILLY ELLIOT (2000): An eleven-year-old boy, son of a coal-mining family, discovers he loves ballet. The sheer exuberance of the kid is inspiring!

STEP UP (2006): Yummy Channing Tatum stars in this bad-boy-turned-good story centered around dancing.

BLACK SWAN (2012): Natalie Portman does a stunning job of portraying a young ballet dancer descending into madness.

MAGIC MIKE (2012): Nothing is more delicious than a hot guy who can dance. Channing Tatum (again!) and Matthew McConaughey steam up the screen in this story of an ambitious male strip club performer.

Chapter 18

Finale

Ginger Rogers did everything that Fred Astaire did. She just did it backwards and in high heels.

—ROBERT THAVES

Congratulations! You've successfully completed your 8-week BBS program.

Now it's time to get the nitty-gritty facts about just what you've accomplished in the last 8 weeks. Remember those measurements and photographs you took a few months ago? Get them back out . . . it's time to do it again. This time, however, the process is probably going to be a little more fun.

Take a new set of pictures of yourself—from the front, side, and back—and measure your hips, thighs, arms, and waist again. Write down your results, then compare them to your originals. What do you see? I bet you've lost several inches over your whole body, and that your new photographs look slamming!

Now for the big test: get out those jeans and put them on. And . . . how do they fit? Are they looser in the waist, bum, and thighs? Do you feel confident and sexy in them? Find an excuse to wear them this weekend, and wear them with pride. You've earned it.

Take this opportunity to write in your journal about how you're feeling right now, so you remember exactly what you've accomplished. You can look back on this entry when you're in need of motivation or inspiration and get all fired up again!

Class Act

Now that you've started dancing, I hope you'll want to continue! There are so many kinds of dance out there, you're sure to find something that suits your tastes. Here is a short list of some of the styles you might like. Go out and take a class or two!

Tap	Break	Jazz	African
Ballet	Krump	Lindy Hop	Salsa
Tango	Swing	Polka	Freestyle
Belly	Square	Tribal	Flamenco
Hip-hop	Folk	Bollywood	Irish Step

Goals, Revisited

Look at the goal you wrote down at the beginning of this program. Did you reach it? If so, good job! But guess what? It's time to make a new goal.

Perhaps you want to lose a few more inches in your waist, or tone up your arms and legs some more in time for summer, or for a vacation. Maybe you want to get even stronger and leaner than you are now. Whatever your new goal, do the same thing you did for your initial one: write it down and think about it each and every day. Set yourself another time limit to accomplish this goal: 8 weeks, 10 weeks, whatever you think is realistic. Then get moving and grooving!

Now, some of you might not have reached the goal that you decided on eight weeks ago. Take a hard look at that goal right now. Is it something achievable? If not, then create a new goal that you know you are capable of reaching and devise a course of action for getting there. If your goal wasn't unrealistic, think about where you might have gone wrong. Not everything works out perfectly all the time, so if your jeans are still snug or you have not lost the inches you were hoping for, don't beat yourself up. Listed below are some factors that might have kept you from meeting your goals. Look to see where you can make improvements and continue the program for several more weeks. After that, assess your progress again.

- SKIPPING WORKOUTS. It's okay to miss a workout every now and then, but if you're consistently skipping your workouts, you might not be ready to make exercise and healthy living a lifestyle. Do a little soul-searching and see where you are on this front.
- SKIPPING PART OF YOUR WORKOUT. It's important to do both the strength and the cardio portions of your workout. Granted, some people love to do one half and don't love doing the other half, but both are important for success.
- BRAIN DRAIN. I know that when I have something on my mind it's difficult for me to shift my full attention onto something else, but I do my best to clear my head and really focus on my workout once I meet with a client or walk into my studio. In fact, I find that if I let the problem lie for an hour while I move my body and focus on something else, when I return to thinking about it, the answer has suddenly appeared! Working out can be a great way to help you get through difficult situations or stressful days. It's never a good idea to skip a workout because you're in a mental slump—working out is the thing that will help shake you out if it!
- LACK OF INTENSITY. This issue can also be a matter of mental focus. If you find your mind wandering when you're training, do your best to bring it back to the present. Concentrate on each repetition or dance step and make it as precise and intense as possible. A lack of intensity can also be a matter of energy; if you have been burning the candle at both ends, you might be overtired and aren't able to give your workouts the energy needed to make them effective. Look back on your journal and evaluate your sleeping and working patterns over the last two months. See where you can make improvements so you can give your workouts 100%.
- MAKING POOR FOOD CHOICES. Remember that what you eat has everything to do with your energy and how you look and feel. If you know you've been making poor food choices over the last 8 weeks, chances are that's the culprit that's derailed you. Look over your journal and see where you can make improvements. Be honest with yourself about what you've been eating. Reread

the "Fuel Your Fire" section (pages 131–188) for ideas on how to improve your eating habits.

- PERSONAL DRAMA. Believe me, I know about drama! And, yes, it's really difficult not to let major life changes derail your program. If during the last 8 weeks you've experienced a huge life change, cut yourself some slack. You'll need time to regroup, so if you haven't met your goal, then so be it. Just remember that exercise can help relieve the stress and depression that can come with such upheavals. Continue to work out, and when you're feeling better, get back on track. This book isn't going anywhere; you can certainly start again when you're ready to dedicate yourself to it fully.

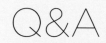

QUESTION: Initially I lost weight and saw changes with BBS, but now I've hit a plateau: I have been hovering at the same weight and size for weeks. Should I work out more? Change my diet?

ANSWER: Even professional athletes hit sticking points in their programs, so you are definitely not alone. But don't take drastic measures to get yourself back on track. Exercising too much can lead to overtraining and possibly injury, and cutting too far back on your food intake can cause your body to store the food you do eat as fat. Chances are your body easily lost a bunch of excess weight at the beginning in the form of fluid, fat, and extra waste. But as you get healthier, it becomes harder to keep losing at a steady pace. The best way to get through your plateau is to increase the intensity and change up the variety of your workouts.

Conclusion

Take a Bow

You have to love dancing to stick to it. It gives you nothing back, no manuscripts to store away, no paintings to show on walls and maybe hang in museums, no poems to be printed and sold, nothing but that single fleeting moment when you feel alive.

—MERCE CUNNINGHAM

So you find yourself at the end of the book—congratulations! You have survived the 8-Week Total-Body-Makeover Plan and have hopefully achieved your goal. My ultimate wish for you is that you've learned a lot about yourself and your capabilities, have challenged yourself both mentally and physically, and that you've come out the other side a happier, more whole person. Remember, we must always push ourselves to achieve bigger and better things—don't be scared and never back down!

Thank you for sharing this journey with me. I hope you now look at exercise and healthful eating as a way of life and not a tedious chore, and that you feel revived, transformed, and ready to conquer all of life's challenges.

Many thanks and remember to—

ALWAYS KEEP ON DANCING!

Much love,

Simone

Acknowledgments

First, I would like to thank my editor, Julie Will, for believing in me and allowing me to write the book I wanted. My co-writer, Lara McGlashan—thank you for capturing my voice and making sense of my crazy dance moves. And many thanks to the talented Zoe Buckman who always makes me feel so comfortable in front of the camera.

To my business partner and friend Grace Hightower De Niro: I am eternally grateful for your support. You allowed my dream to become a reality. I love you, darling!

Thank you also to my longest living friend and "adopted brother" Gerrard Carter, who always reminds me of the power of laughter (especially at oneself!), and to my best girlfriend and Barbie partner-in-crime Deone Zanotto, who centers me and has been by my side for this crazy journey.

To my fabulous team of trainers at BBS: without you I would be nothing. Your beautiful energy and spirits are what make BBS so special.

To my clients: You inspire me every day to push and strive for perfection. A special thank-you to my original clients Chelsea, Lucy, Grace, Zoe, Sandy, Naomi, and Annie who have been with me since the beginning. You have followed me from hired ballroom dance studios to shoebox apartments and now, finally, to my NYC and LA studios. Your loyalty and friendship means the world.

And finally, to my darling mother who is my everything. Every day you teach me to be a better woman. Thank you.

Index

About the Author

Simone De La Rue began training in classical ballet at the age of three and has enjoyed a successful dance career spanning two decades, including numerous performances on Broadway, London's West End, and in her native Australia. She is the creator and owner of BODY BY SIMONE technique and currently has two studios in New York City and Los Angeles.